DIET & FITNESS JOURNAL

This journal belongs to

The difference between a dream and a reality
is the action we take in between.

PERSONAL PROFILE

Age: _____

Weight: _____

Height: _____

Describe your body type.

_____

_____

_____

_____

_____

Which body area are you most proud of?

_____

_____

_____

_____

_____

Which body area would you like to see the most improved?

_____

_____

_____

_____

Calculate your body mass index (BMI):

Body mass index (BMI) is one of many ways to measure body fat based on your height and weight. The calculation below can indicate if you are underweight, normal, overweight, or obese. Use the calculation or chart below to assess your body mass index, then use this number as a starting point for this diet and fitness journal.

Current BMI range: _____

Desired BMI range: _____

$$\frac{\text{weight in pounds}}{\text{(height in inches} \times \text{height in inches)}} \times 703 = BMI$$

BMI	19	20	21	22	23	24	25	26	27	28	29	30	35	40
						WEIGHT								
4'10"	91	96	100	105	110	115	119	124	129	134	138	143	167	191
4'11"	94	99	104	109	114	119	124	128	133	138	143	148	173	198
5'0"	97	102	107	112	118	123	128	133	138	143	148	153	179	204
5'1"	100	106	111	116	122	127	132	137	143	148	153	158	185	211
5'2"	104	109	115	120	126	131	136	142	147	153	158	164	191	218
5'3"	107	113	118	124	130	135	141	146	152	158	163	169	197	225
5'4"	110	116	122	128	134	140	145	151	157	163	169	174	204	232
5'5"	114	120	126	132	138	144	150	156	162	168	174	180	210	240
5'6"	118	124	130	136	142	148	155	161	167	173	179	186	216	247
5'7"	121	127	134	140	146	153	159	166	172	178	185	191	223	255
5'8"	125	131	138	144	151	158	164	171	177	184	190	197	230	262
5'9"	128	135	142	149	155	162	169	176	182	189	196	203	236	270
5'10"	132	139	146	153	160	167	174	181	188	195	202	207	243	278
5'11"	136	143	150	157	165	172	179	186	193	200	208	215	250	286
6'0"	140	147	154	162	169	177	184	191	199	206	213	221	258	294
6'1"	144	151	159	166	174	182	189	197	204	212	219	227	265	302
6'2"	148	155	163	171	179	186	194	202	210	218	225	233	272	311
6'3"	152	160	168	176	184	192	200	208	216	224	232	240	279	319
6'4"	156	164	172	180	189	197	205	213	221	230	238	246	287	328

HEIGHT

18.5 or less. . . . . Underweight
18.5 to 24.99. . . . . Normal Weight
25 to 29.99. . . . . Overweight

30 to 34.99. . . . . Obesity (Class 1)
35 to 39.99. . . . . Obesity (Class 2)
40 or greater . . . . Morbid Obesity

Source: Evidence Report of Clinical Guidelines on the Identification, Evaluation, and Treatment of Overweight and Obesity in Adults, 1998. NIH/National Heart, Lung, and Blood Institute (NHLBI)

MY GOALS

How much weight do you want to lose? _____

Is there a specific health goal you would like to meet?

- [ ] Lose over 25 pounds
- [ ] Lose a small amount of weight
- [ ] Maintain current weight
- [ ] Improve muscle tone
- [ ] Decrease fat
- [ ] Improve endurance
- [ ] _____
- [ ] _____

What made you decide to keep a diet and fitness journal?

_____

_____

_____

Is there an event you would like to lose weight for?

_____

_____

_____

Is there a piece of clothing or an outfit you'd like to fit into?

_____

_____

_____

Before Photo
Weight at time of photo: _____ Date: _____

After Photo
Weight at time of photo: _____ Date: _____

My Inspiration

What is your inspiration for keeping this journal?

_____

_____

_____

_____

_____

_____

_____

Is there anyone who inspires you to meet your diet and fitness goals?

_____

_____

_____

_____

_____

_____

_____

_____

_____

When did you make the decision to keep this journal?

_____

_____

_____

_____

_____

_____

_____

_____

Who will be supporting you throughout this process?

_____

_____

_____

_____

_____

_____

_____

_____

_____

_____

GAME PLAN

What is the first step to change my daily diet & fitness routine?

_____

_____

_____

_____

_____

Is there a specific food or calorie plan I am going to follow?

_____

_____

_____

_____

_____

What is my exercise plan?

_____

_____

_____

_____

_____

One thing I'm looking forward to:

_____

_____

_____

_____

_____

_____

One thing I'm dreading:

_____

_____

_____

_____

_____

The people I can call for support are :

_____

_____

_____

_____

_____

WEBSITES & PASSWORDS

Please use this page to record any websites and passwords that you are using while completing this journal.

Website: _____

Password: _____

How will this website help you achieve your goals?

_____

_____

Which part of this website is the most helpful?

_____

_____

_____

Website: _____

Password: _____

How will this website help you achieve your goals?

_____

_____

Which part of this website is the most helpful?

_____

_____

_____

Website: _____

Password: _____

How will this website help you achieve your goals?

_____

_____

_____

Which part of this website is the most helpful?

_____

_____

_____

Website: _____

Password: _____

How will this website help you achieve your goals?

_____

_____

_____

Which part of this website is the most helpful?

_____

_____

_____

TEN USEFUL TIPS

Refer to these pages for quick tips on diet and exercise.

1. Drink Water:

- Drinking up to 8 glasses of water a day will help keep you hydrated and benefit your weight loss efforts. Water can also help you fill up before you eat. One big glass of water before each meal can help you feel more full, so you won't be tempted to overeat.

2. Go For a Walk:

- Invest in a pedometer and try to walk 10,000 steps each day. Simple changes like skipping the elevator and taking the stairs or parking in the back of the lot will help you add up extra steps.

3. Lighten Up:

- Lessen your calorie count by swapping out a few things in your kitchen: Swap 2% milk for skim milk, bake with applesauce instead of oil, eat low-fat cheese instead of full-fat cheese, try baked chips instead of fried chips, ditch high-calorie sodas for seltzers with a twist of lime or lemon.

4. Time Out:

- Eat meals and snacks at the same time every day. You won't be as tempted to graze on extra food if you know exactly when you will have your next meal or snack.

5. Take It To the Table:

- Eat meals at a table away from your TV or computer to avoid eating too quickly and going back for seconds. Instead of watching TV, you'll be watching what you eat.

6. Whole Grains:

- White bread and pasta are filled with carbohydrates and little nutrients. Try cooking with whole-grain or whole-wheat breads and pastas that contain fiber and protein.

7. Freeze Out:

- Keeping your freezer stocked with frozen fruits, veggies, and leftovers can help create healthy meals in a flash. Instead of turning to the phone for take-out, open up your freezer and defrost a healthy meal in less than half the time it'll take that pizza delivery to reach your door.

8. Buddy Up:

- Finding motivation to keep up with your diet and exercise routine on your own can be tough. Working out and dieting with a friend can help keep you both on track!

9. Portion Control:

- At home, use smaller salad plates instead of large dinner plates for each meal. This way you can fill up your plate, and not your waistline.

10. Get Real:

- Set realistic, smaller goals instead of large, overwhelming goals. Large goals are intimidating, and slow progress towards large goals makes it tempting to give up. Instead of making a goal to lose 15 pounds, make a goal to lose 5. After you have reached your 5-pound goal, set another goal to lose an additional 5 pounds.

HOW TO USE THIS JOURNAL

Use this page as a guide for recording your food and exercise routine each week. This journal includes pages for daily entries, followed by a weekly wrap-up.

S M T W R F (S) date **January 7** week # **1**

TODAY'S GOAL MET	FOOD LOG	calories	fat (g)	protein (g)	carbs (g)	fiber
X	**Breakfast** time: 8 am	78	5	6	0	0
	1 hard boiled egg, 1 English muffin,	134	1	4	26	2
	2 tbsp. peanut butter, 2 coffees	190	16	8	7	2
		4	0	1	0	0
MOOD ☹ 2 3 4 ☺	**Snack** time: 10:30 am					
	10 baby carrots, water	40	tr	1	10	1
	Lunch time: 12:30 pm	250	--	--	--	--
	1 tuna fish sandwich, 1 bag baked chips	120	2	2	23	2
	Snack time: 3:30 pm	105	8	4	3	2
	1/8 cup almonds, 1/4 cups raisins	85	--	1	22	2
ENERGY LEVEL	**Dinner** time: 7 pm	368	18	46	0	0
	grilled Salmon, 1 cup brown rice,	216	2	5	45	4
	8 asparagus spears	26	1	2	4	2
2 3 (4)	**Snack** time: 10:30 pm	116	4	3	18	2
	1/2 cup low-fat frozen yogurt with berries	41	1	1	1	1

NUTRIENT TRACKER:			DAILY TOTALS:	
	# of servings	recommended		
WATER	X X X X X X X	8		
FRUITS	X X	2-4	calories	**1,773**
VEGETABLES	X X X	3-5		
GRAINS	X X X X	6-8	carbs **159**	fat **5(**
PROTEIN	X X X X X	3-4		
DAIRY	X	2-3		
SUGARS	X FATS X	moderation	protein **81**	fiber **1(**
VITAMINS/SUPPLEMENTS				

PHYSICAL ACTIVITY	focus	intensity	t
walking on beach	cardio	high	45
gardening	arms	moderate	30

WORKOUT RATE
great
good **X**
okay
meh
missed

COMMENTS/THOUGHTS

I ate a lot of protein today, maybe that's why my energy level was higher than usual.

As you complete each weekly wrap-up, assess your progress from the past week, and set new goals for the week to come.

EEKLY WRAP-UP date *January 7* week # *1*

To be strong is to be happy.
-Longfellow

START WEIGHT
159

END WEIGHT
158

'S I TRACKED MY DIET S X M X T X W X R X F X S X
ET NOTES

Did well this week! Need to concentrate more on portion control and fitting more fruits and vegetables into my diet.

THIS WEEK'S MOOD
☹
2
3
(4)
☺

'S I EXERCISED S M X T W X R X F S X
ERCISE NOTES

45 minutes of cardio is TOUGH!
Proud of myself for plugging through
the last 10 minutes.

THIS WEEK'S ENERGY LEVEL
🐌
2
(3)
4
🐇

Did I meet this week's goals?

%	25%	50%	75%	100%
		X		

TOTAL WORKOUT TIME
3:15

ALS FOR NEXT WEEK

Take a walk before work 2 days next week.

YOU CAN DO THIS!

S M T W R F S

date   week #

	FOOD LOG	calories	fat (g)	protein (g)	carbs (g)	fiber (g)
TODAY'S GOAL MET	**Breakfast** time:					
MOOD ☹ 2 3 4 ☺	**Snack** time:					
	Lunch time:					
	Snack time:					
ENERGY LEVEL 🐌 2 3 4 🐇	**Dinner** time:					
	Snack time:					

NUTRIENT TRACKER:

	# of servings	recommended
WATER		8
FRUITS		2-4
VEGETABLES		3-5
GRAINS		6-8
PROTEIN		3-4
DAIRY		2-3
SUGARS	FATS	moderation
VITAMINS/SUPPLEMENTS		

DAILY TOTALS:

calories

carbs   fat

protein   fiber

WORKOUT RATE

great

good

okay

meh

missed

PHYSICAL ACTIVITY	focus	intensity	tir

COMMENTS/THOUGHTS

M T W R F S   date   week #

FOOD LOG

	calories	fat (g)	protein (g)	carbs (g)	fiber (g)		TODAY'S GOAL MET
breakfast time:							
snack time:							MOOD ☹
lunch time:							2 3 4
snack time:							☺
dinner time:							ENERGY LEVEL 🐌
snack time:							2 3 4 🐇

NUTRIENT TRACKER:

	# of servings	recommended
WATER		8
FRUITS		2-4
VEGETABLES		3-5
GRAINS		6-8
PROTEIN		3-4
DAIRY		2-3
SUGARS	FATS	moderation
VITAMINS/SUPPLEMENTS		

DAILY TOTALS:

calories

carbs   fat

protein   fiber

WORKOUT RATE
great
good
okay
meh
missed

PHYSICAL ACTIVITY

	focus	intensity	time

COMMENTS/THOUGHTS

S M T W R F S   date _____   week # ____

TODAY'S GOAL MET	FOOD LOG	calories	fat (g)	protein (g)	carbs (g)	fiber (g)
	Breakfast time:					
MOOD ☹ 2 3 4 ☺	**Snack** time:					
	Lunch time:					
	Snack time:					
ENERGY LEVEL 🐌 2 3 4 🐇	**Dinner** time:					
	Snack time:					

NUTRIENT TRACKER:

	# of servings	recommended
WATER		8
FRUITS		2-4
VEGETABLES		3-5
GRAINS		6-8
PROTEIN		3-4
DAIRY		2-3
SUGARS	FATS	moderation
VITAMINS/SUPPLEMENTS		

DAILY TOTALS:

calories

carbs   fat

protein   fiber

WORKOUT RATE

great

good

okay

meh

missed

PHYSICAL ACTIVITY	focus	intensity	tir

COMMENTS/THOUGHTS

M T W R F S   date   week #

FOOD LOG

		calories	fat (g)	protein (g)	carbs (g)	fiber (g)	
breakfast time:							
snack time:							
lunch time:							
snack time:							
dinner time:							
snack time:							

TODAY'S GOAL MET

MOOD
☹
2
3
4
☺

ENERGY LEVEL
🐌
2
3
4
🐇

NUTRIENT TRACKER:

	# of servings	recommended
WATER		8
FRUITS		2-4
VEGETABLES		3-5
GRAINS		6-8
PROTEIN		3-4
DAIRY		2-3
SUGARS	FATS	moderation
VITAMINS/SUPPLEMENTS		

DAILY TOTALS:

calories

carbs   fat

protein   fiber

WORKOUT RATE
great
good
okay
meh
missed

PHYSICAL ACTIVITY

	focus	intensity	time

COMMENTS/THOUGHTS

S M T W R F S date week

FOOD LOG

	calories	fat (g)	protein (g)	carbs (g)	fiber (g)
TODAY'S GOAL MET					

Breakfast
time:

MOOD
☹
2
3
4
☺

Snack
time:

Lunch
time:

Snack
time:

ENERGY LEVEL
🐌
2
3
4
🐇

Dinner
time:

Snack
time:

NUTRIENT TRACKER:

	# of servings	recommended
WATER		8
FRUITS		2-4
VEGETABLES		3-5
GRAINS		6-8
PROTEIN		3-4
DAIRY		2-3
SUGARS	FATS	moderation
VITAMINS/SUPPLEMENTS		

DAILY TOTALS:

calories

carbs   fat

protein   fiber

WORKOUT RATE

great

good

okay

meh

missed

PHYSICAL ACTIVITY

	focus	intensity	tim

COMMENTS/THOUGHTS

M T W R F S   date [   ]   week # [   ]

FOOD LOG

	calories	fat (g)	protein (g)	carbs (g)	fiber (g)	
breakfast time:						
snack time:						
lunch time:						
snack time:						
dinner time:						
snack time:						

TODAY'S GOAL MET

MOOD
☹
2
3
4
☺

ENERGY LEVEL
🐌
2
3
4
🐇

NUTRIENT TRACKER:

	# of servings	recommended
WATER		8
FRUITS		2-4
VEGETABLES		3-5
GRAINS		6-8
PROTEIN		3-4
DAIRY		2-3
SUGARS	FATS	moderation
VITAMINS/SUPPLEMENTS		

DAILY TOTALS:

calories

carbs   fat

protein   fiber

WORKOUT RATE
great
good
okay
meh
missed

PHYSICAL ACTIVITY

	focus	intensity	time

COMMENTS/THOUGHTS

S M T W R F S   date _____   week # _____

TODAY'S GOAL MET	FOOD LOG	calories	fat (g)	protein (g)	carbs (g)	fiber (g)
	Breakfast time:					
MOOD ☹ 2 3 4 ☺	**Snack** time:					
	Lunch time:					
	Snack time:					
ENERGY LEVEL 🐌 2 3 4 🐇	**Dinner** time:					
	Snack time:					

NUTRIENT TRACKER:

	# of servings	recommended
WATER		8
FRUITS		2-4
VEGETABLES		3-5
GRAINS		6-8
PROTEIN		3-4
DAIRY		2-3
SUGARS	FATS	moderation
VITAMINS/SUPPLEMENTS		

DAILY TOTALS:

calories _____

carbs _____   fat _____

protein _____   fiber _____

WORKOUT RATE	PHYSICAL ACTIVITY	focus	intensity	tin
great				
good				
okay				
meh				
missed				

COMMENTS/THOUGHTS

WEEKLY WRAP-UP

date   week #

	START WEIGHT

To be strong is to be happy.
-Longfellow

END WEIGHT

AYS I TRACKED MY DIET   S   M   T   W   R   F   S

IET NOTES

THIS WEEK'S MOOD

☹

2

3

4

☺

AYS I EXERCISED   S   M   T   W   R   F   S

XERCISE NOTES

THIS WEEK'S ENERGY LEVEL

🐌

2

3

4

🐇

Did I meet this week's goals?

0%   25%   50%   75%   100%

TOTAL WORKOUT TIME

OALS FOR NEXT WEEK

YOU CAN DO THIS!

S M T W R F S   date ___   week # ___

FOOD LOG

	calories	fat (g)	protein (g)	carbs (g)	fiber (g)
Breakfast time:					
Snack time:					
Lunch time:					
Snack time:					
Dinner time:					
Snack time:					

TODAY'S GOAL MET

MOOD
☹ 2 3 4 ☺

ENERGY LEVEL
🐌 2 3 4 🐇

WORKOUT RATE
great
good
okay
meh
missed

NUTRIENT TRACKER:

	# of servings	recommended
WATER		8
FRUITS		2-4
VEGETABLES		3-5
GRAINS		6-8
PROTEIN		3-4
DAIRY		2-3
SUGARS	FATS	moderation
VITAMINS/SUPPLEMENTS		

DAILY TOTALS:

calories

carbs | fat

protein | fiber

PHYSICAL ACTIVITY

	focus	intensity	tim

COMMENTS/THOUGHTS

M T W R F S   date _____   week # _____

FOOD LOG

	calories	fat (g)	protein (g)	carbs (g)	fiber (g)
breakfast time:					
snack time:					
lunch time:					
snack time:					
dinner time:					
snack time:					

TODAY'S GOAL MET

MOOD

☹
2
3
4
☺

ENERGY LEVEL

🐌
2
3
4
🐇

WORKOUT RATE

great

good

okay

meh

missed

NUTRIENT TRACKER:

	# of servings	recommended
WATER		8
FRUITS		2-4
VEGETABLES		3-5
GRAINS		6-8
PROTEIN		3-4
DAIRY		2-3
SUGARS	FATS	moderation
VITAMINS/SUPPLEMENTS		

DAILY TOTALS:

calories

carbs   fat

protein   fiber

PHYSICAL ACTIVITY

	focus	intensity	time

COMMENTS/THOUGHTS

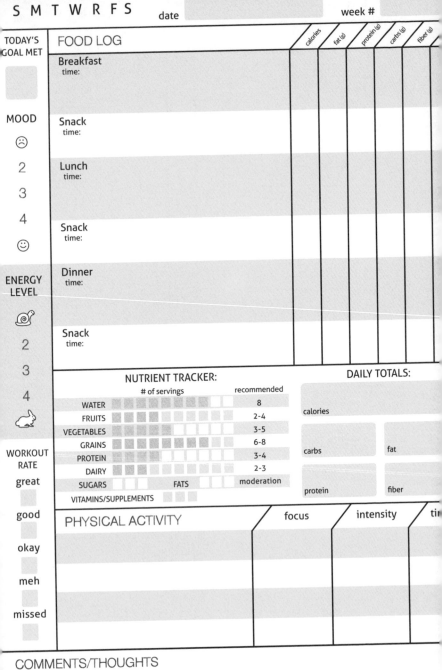

S M T W R F S date week #

TODAY'S GOAL MET	FOOD LOG	calories	fat (g)	protein (g)	carbs (g)	fiber (g)
	Breakfast time:					
MOOD ☹ 2 3 4 ☺	**Snack** time:					
	Lunch time:					
	Snack time:					
ENERGY LEVEL 🐌 2 3 4 🐇	**Dinner** time:					
	Snack time:					

NUTRIENT TRACKER:

	# of servings	recommended
WATER		8
FRUITS		2-4
VEGETABLES		3-5
GRAINS		6-8
PROTEIN		3-4
DAIRY		2-3
SUGARS	FATS	moderation
VITAMINS/SUPPLEMENTS		

DAILY TOTALS:

calories

carbs   fat

protein   fiber

WORKOUT RATE
great
good
okay
meh
missed

PHYSICAL ACTIVITY	focus	intensity	ti

COMMENTS/THOUGHTS

M T W R F S   date   week #

FOOD LOG

	calories	fat (g)	protein (g)	carbs (g)	fiber (g)
breakfast time:					
snack time:					
lunch time:					
snack time:					
dinner time:					
snack time:					

TODAY'S GOAL MET

MOOD

☹
2
3
4
☺

ENERGY LEVEL

🐌
2
3
4
🐰

NUTRIENT TRACKER:

	# of servings	recommended
WATER		8
FRUITS		2-4
VEGETABLES		3-5
GRAINS		6-8
PROTEIN		3-4
DAIRY		2-3
SUGARS	FATS	moderation
VITAMINS/SUPPLEMENTS		

DAILY TOTALS:

calories

carbs   fat

protein   fiber

WORKOUT RATE

great

good

okay

meh

missed

PHYSICAL ACTIVITY

	focus	intensity	time

COMMENTS/THOUGHTS

S M T W R F S   date   week #

TODAY'S GOAL MET	FOOD LOG	calories	fat (g)	protein (g)	carbs (g)	fiber (g)
	Breakfast time:					
MOOD ☹ 2 3 4 ☺	**Snack** time:					
	Lunch time:					
	Snack time:					
ENERGY LEVEL 🐌 2 3 4 🐇	**Dinner** time:					
	Snack time:					

NUTRIENT TRACKER:

	# of servings	recommended
WATER		8
FRUITS		2-4
VEGETABLES		3-5
GRAINS		6-8
PROTEIN		3-4
DAIRY		2-3
SUGARS	FATS	moderation
VITAMINS/SUPPLEMENTS		

DAILY TOTALS:

calories

carbs   fat

protein   fiber

WORKOUT RATE	PHYSICAL ACTIVITY	focus	intensity	time
great				
good				
okay				
meh				
missed				

COMMENTS/THOUGHTS

M T W R F S

date _____ week # _____

FOOD LOG

	calories	fat (g)	protein (g)	carbs (g)	fiber (g)	
Breakfast time:						
Snack time:						
Lunch time:						
Snack time:						
Dinner time:						
Snack time:						

TODAY'S GOAL MET

MOOD

☹
2
3
4
☺

ENERGY LEVEL

🐌
2
3
4
🐇

NUTRIENT TRACKER:

	# of servings	recommended
WATER		8
FRUITS		2-4
VEGETABLES		3-5
GRAINS		6-8
PROTEIN		3-4
DAIRY		2-3
SUGARS	FATS	moderation
VITAMINS/SUPPLEMENTS		

DAILY TOTALS:

calories

carbs

fat

protein

fiber

WORKOUT RATE

great

good

okay

meh

missed

PHYSICAL ACTIVITY

	focus	intensity	time

COMMENTS/THOUGHTS

S M T W R F S

date   week #

TODAY'S GOAL MET	FOOD LOG	calories	fat (g)	protein (g)	carbs (g)	fiber (g)
	Breakfast time:					
MOOD ☹ 2 3 4 ☺	**Snack** time:					
	Lunch time:					
	Snack time:					
ENERGY LEVEL 🐌 2 3 4 🐇	**Dinner** time:					
	Snack time:					

NUTRIENT TRACKER:

	# of servings	recommended
WATER		8
FRUITS		2-4
VEGETABLES		3-5
GRAINS		6-8
PROTEIN		3-4
DAIRY		2-3
SUGARS	FATS	moderation
VITAMINS/SUPPLEMENTS		

DAILY TOTALS:

calories

carbs   fat

protein   fiber

WORKOUT RATE

great

good

okay

meh

missed

PHYSICAL ACTIVITY	focus	intensity	tir

COMMENTS/THOUGHTS

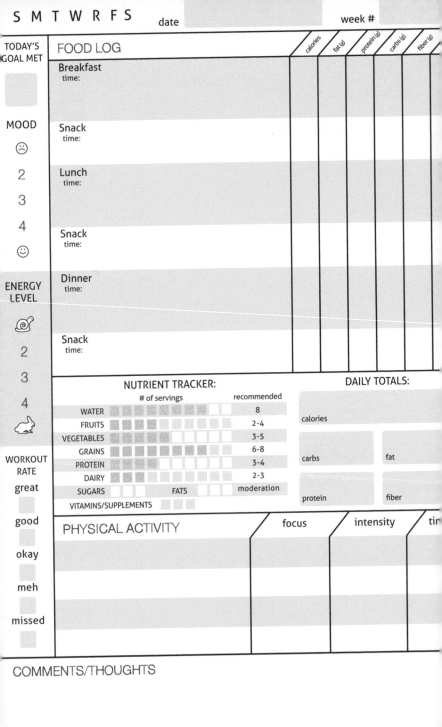

WEEKLY WRAP-UP

date _____   week # _____

| | START WEIGHT |
| | END WEIGHT |

Patience and fortitude conquer all things.

-Emerson

DAYS I TRACKED MY DIET   S ☐ M ☐ T ☐ W ☐ R ☐ F ☐ S ☐

DIET NOTES

THIS WEEK'S MOOD

☹

2

3

4

☺

DAYS I EXERCISED   S ☐ M ☐ T ☐ W ☐ R ☐ F ☐ S ☐

EXERCISE NOTES

THIS WEEK'S ENERGY LEVEL

🐌

2

3

4

🐇

Did I meet this week's goals?

0%   25%   50%   75%   100%

TOTAL WORKOUT TIME

GOALS FOR NEXT WEEK

YOU CAN DO THIS!

S M T W R F S   date   week

TODAY'S GOAL MET

FOOD LOG

	calories	fat (g)	protein (g)	carbs (g)	fiber (g)
Breakfast time:					
Snack time:					
Lunch time:					
Snack time:					
Dinner time:					
Snack time:					

MOOD

☹
2
3
4
☺

ENERGY LEVEL

🐌
2
3
4
🐇

NUTRIENT TRACKER:

	# of servings	recommended
WATER		8
FRUITS		2-4
VEGETABLES		3-5
GRAINS		6-8
PROTEIN		3-4
DAIRY		2-3
SUGARS	FATS	moderation
VITAMINS/SUPPLEMENTS		

DAILY TOTALS:

calories

carbs

fat

protein

fiber

WORKOUT RATE

great

good

okay

meh

missed

PHYSICAL ACTIVITY

	focus	intensity	tir

COMMENTS/THOUGHTS

M T W R F S   date   week #

OOD LOG

	calories	fat (g)	protein (g)	carbs (g)	fiber (g)		TODAY'S GOAL MET
eakfast ne:							
ack ne:							**MOOD**
nch ne:							☹ 2 3 4 ☺
ack ne:							
nner ne:							**ENERGY LEVEL**
ack ne:							

NUTRIENT TRACKER:

	# of servings	recommended
WATER		8
FRUITS		2-4
ABLES		3-5
RAINS		6-8
ROTEIN		3-4
DAIRY		2-3
GARS	FATS	moderation
MINS/SUPPLEMENTS		

DAILY TOTALS:

calories

carbs   fat

protein   fiber

ENERGY LEVEL

🐌 2 3 4 🐇

WORKOUT RATE
great
good
okay
meh
missed

YSICAL ACTIVITY	focus	intensity	time

OMMENTS/THOUGHTS

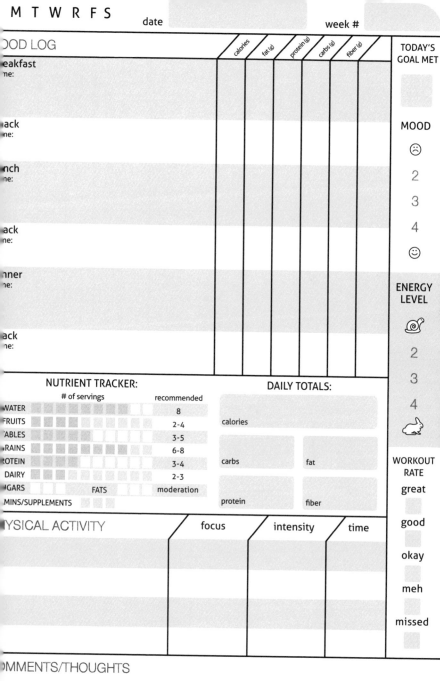

S M T W R F S date   week #

TODAY'S GOAL MET	FOOD LOG	calories	fat (g)	protein (g)	carbs (g)	fiber (g)
	Breakfast time:					
MOOD ☹ 2 3 4 ☺	**Snack** time:					
	Lunch time:					
	Snack time:					
ENERGY LEVEL 🐌 2 3 4 🐇	**Dinner** time:					
	Snack time:					

NUTRIENT TRACKER:

	# of servings	recommended
WATER		8
FRUITS		2-4
VEGETABLES		3-5
GRAINS		6-8
PROTEIN		3-4
DAIRY		2-3
SUGARS	FATS	moderation
VITAMINS/SUPPLEMENTS		

DAILY TOTALS:

calories

carbs   fat

protein   fiber

WORKOUT RATE

great

good

okay

meh

missed

PHYSICAL ACTIVITY	focus	intensity	ti

COMMENTS/THOUGHTS

M T W R F S   date   week #

OOD LOG

	calories	fat (g)	protein (g)	carbs (g)	fiber (g)
reakfast ime:					
nack me:					
unch me:					
ack me:					
nner me:					
ack me:					

TODAY'S GOAL MET

MOOD

☹

2

3

4

☺

ENERGY LEVEL

🐌

2

3

4

🐇

WORKOUT RATE

great

good

okay

meh

missed

NUTRIENT TRACKER:

	# of servings	recommended
WATER		8
FRUITS		2-4
TABLES		3-5
GRAINS		6-8
ROTEIN		3-4
DAIRY		2-3
UGARS	FATS	moderation
AMINS/SUPPLEMENTS		

DAILY TOTALS:

calories

carbs

fat

protein

fiber

HYSICAL ACTIVITY	focus	intensity	time

OMMENTS/THOUGHTS

S M T W R F S

date   week #

TODAY'S GOAL MET	FOOD LOG	calories	fat (g)	protein (g)	carbs (g)	fiber (g)
	Breakfast time:					
MOOD ☹ 2 3 4 ☺	**Snack** time:					
	Lunch time:					
	Snack time:					
ENERGY LEVEL 🐌 2 3 4 🐇	**Dinner** time:					
	Snack time:					

NUTRIENT TRACKER:

	# of servings	recommended
WATER		8
FRUITS		2-4
VEGETABLES		3-5
GRAINS		6-8
PROTEIN		3-4
DAIRY		2-3
SUGARS	FATS	moderation
VITAMINS/SUPPLEMENTS		

DAILY TOTALS:

calories

carbs   fat

protein   fiber

WORKOUT RATE

great

good

okay

meh

missed

PHYSICAL ACTIVITY	focus	intensity	tir

COMMENTS/THOUGHTS

M T W R F S date _____ week # _____

FOOD LOG

	calories	fat (g)	protein (g)	carbs (g)	fiber (g)	
Breakfast time:						
Snack time:						
Lunch time:						
Snack time:						
Dinner time:						
Snack time:						

NUTRIENT TRACKER:

	# of servings	recommended
WATER		8
FRUITS		2-4
VEGETABLES		3-5
GRAINS		6-8
PROTEIN		3-4
DAIRY		2-3
SUGARS	FATS	moderation
VITAMINS/SUPPLEMENTS		

DAILY TOTALS:

calories _____

carbs _____   fat _____

protein _____   fiber _____

PHYSICAL ACTIVITY

	focus	intensity	time

TODAY'S GOAL MET

MOOD
☹
2
3
4
☺

ENERGY LEVEL
🐌
2
3
4
🐇

WORKOUT RATE
great
good
okay
meh
missed

COMMENTS/THOUGHTS

S M T W R F S   date   week #

TODAY'S GOAL MET	FOOD LOG	calories	fat (g)	protein (g)	carbs (g)	fiber (g)
	Breakfast time:					
MOOD ☹ 2 3 4 ☺	**Snack** time:					
	Lunch time:					
	Snack time:					
ENERGY LEVEL 🐌 2 3 4 🐰	**Dinner** time:					
	Snack time:					

NUTRIENT TRACKER:

	# of servings	recommended
WATER		8
FRUITS		2-4
VEGETABLES		3-5
GRAINS		6-8
PROTEIN		3-4
DAIRY		2-3
SUGARS	FATS	moderation
VITAMINS/SUPPLEMENTS		

DAILY TOTALS:

calories

carbs   fat

protein   fiber

WORKOUT RATE	PHYSICAL ACTIVITY	focus	intensity	tim
great				
good				
okay				
meh				
missed				

COMMENTS/THOUGHTS

START WEIGHT

Whatever is worth doing at all,
is worth doing well.

-Earl of Chesterfield

END WEIGHT

DAYS I TRACKED MY DIET   S   M   T   W   R   F   S

DIET NOTES

THIS WEEK'S MOOD

☹

2

3

4

☺

DAYS I EXERCISED   S   M   T   W   R   F   S

EXERCISE NOTES

THIS WEEK'S ENERGY LEVEL

🐌

2

3

4

🐇

Did I meet this week's goals?

TOTAL WORKOUT TIME

0%   25%   50%   75%   100%

GOALS FOR NEXT WEEK

YOU CAN DO THIS!

S M T W R F S

date

week #

TODAY'S GOAL MET

FOOD LOG

	calories	fat (g)	protein (g)	carbs (g)	fiber (g)
Breakfast time:					
Snack time:					
Lunch time:					
Snack time:					
Dinner time:					
Snack time:					

MOOD

☹
2
3
4
☺

ENERGY LEVEL

🐌
2
3
4
🐰

NUTRIENT TRACKER:

	# of servings	recommended
WATER		8
FRUITS		2-4
VEGETABLES		3-5
GRAINS		6-8
PROTEIN		3-4
DAIRY		2-3
SUGARS	FATS	moderation
VITAMINS/SUPPLEMENTS		

DAILY TOTALS:

calories

carbs   fat

protein   fiber

WORKOUT RATE

great
good
okay
meh
missed

PHYSICAL ACTIVITY

	focus	intensity	tir

COMMENTS/THOUGHTS

M T W R F S   date   week #

OOD LOG

	calories	fat (g)	protein (g)	carbs (g)	fiber (g)	

reakfast
ime:

nack
ime:

unch
ime:

nack
ime:

inner
ime:

nack
ime:

NUTRIENT TRACKER:

	# of servings	recommended
WATER		8
FRUITS		2-4
ETABLES		3-5
GRAINS		6-8
PROTEIN		3-4
DAIRY		2-3
SUGARS	FATS	moderation
AMINS/SUPPLEMENTS		

DAILY TOTALS:

calories

carbs   fat

protein   fiber

HYSICAL ACTIVITY

	focus	intensity	time

TODAY'S GOAL MET

MOOD

☹

2

3

4

☺

ENERGY LEVEL

🐌

2

3

4

🐇

WORKOUT RATE

great

good

okay

meh

missed

OMMENTS/THOUGHTS

S M T W R F S   date   week #

	FOOD LOG	calories	fat (g)	protein (g)	carbs (g)	fiber (g)
TODAY'S GOAL MET	**Breakfast** time:					
MOOD ☹ 2 3 4 ☺	**Snack** time:					
	Lunch time:					
	Snack time:					
ENERGY LEVEL 🐌 2 3 4 🐰	**Dinner** time:					
	Snack time:					

NUTRIENT TRACKER:

	# of servings	recommended
WATER		8
FRUITS		2-4
VEGETABLES		3-5
GRAINS		6-8
PROTEIN		3-4
DAIRY		2-3
SUGARS	FATS	moderation
VITAMINS/SUPPLEMENTS		

DAILY TOTALS:

calories

carbs   fat

protein   fiber

WORKOUT RATE

great

good

okay

meh

missed

PHYSICAL ACTIVITY	focus	intensity	tim

COMMENTS/THOUGHTS

M T W R F S

date _____ week # _____

[F]OOD LOG

	calories	fat (g)	protein (g)	carbs (g)	fiber (g)		
[Br]eakfast [ti]me:							
[Sn]ack [ti]me:							
[Lu]nch [ti]me:							
[Sn]ack [ti]me:							
[Di]nner [ti]me:							
[Sn]ack [ti]me:							

NUTRIENT TRACKER:

	# of servings	recommended
[W]ATER		8
[F]RUITS		2-4
[VEGE]TABLES		3-5
[G]RAINS		6-8
[PR]OTEIN		3-4
DAIRY		2-3
[S]UGARS	FATS	moderation
[VIT]AMINS/SUPPLEMENTS		

DAILY TOTALS:

calories

carbs   fat

protein   fiber

[PH]YSICAL ACTIVITY

	focus	intensity	time

[CO]MMENTS/THOUGHTS

TODAY'S GOAL MET

MOOD
🙁
2
3
4
🙂

ENERGY LEVEL
🐌
2
3
4
🐰

WORKOUT RATE
great

good

okay

meh

missed

S M T W R F S   date   week

TODAY'S GOAL MET	FOOD LOG	calories	fat (g)	protein (g)	carbs (g)	fiber (g)
	Breakfast time:					
MOOD ☹ 2 3 4 ☺	**Snack** time:					
	Lunch time:					
	Snack time:					
ENERGY LEVEL 🐌 2 3 4 🐇	**Dinner** time:					
	Snack time:					

NUTRIENT TRACKER:

	# of servings	recommended
WATER		8
FRUITS		2-4
VEGETABLES		3-5
GRAINS		6-8
PROTEIN		3-4
DAIRY		2-3
SUGARS	FATS	moderation
VITAMINS/SUPPLEMENTS		

DAILY TOTALS:

calories

carbs   fat

protein   fiber

WORKOUT RATE	PHYSICAL ACTIVITY	focus	intensity	ti...
great				
good				
okay				
meh				
missed				

COMMENTS/THOUGHTS

M T W R F S

date   week #

OOD LOG

	calories	fat (g)	protein (g)	carbs (g)	fiber (g)
eakfast ne:					
ack ne:					
nch ne:					
ack ne:					
nner ne:					
ack ne:					

TODAY'S GOAL MET

MOOD

☹
2
3
4
☺

ENERGY LEVEL

🐌
2
3
4
🐰

NUTRIENT TRACKER:

	# of servings	recommended
WATER		8
FRUITS		2-4
TABLES		3-5
GRAINS		6-8
ROTEIN		3-4
DAIRY		2-3
UGARS	FATS	moderation
MINS/SUPPLEMENTS		

DAILY TOTALS:

calories

carbs   fat

protein   fiber

WORKOUT RATE

great

good

okay

meh

missed

HYSICAL ACTIVITY

	focus	intensity	time

OMMENTS/THOUGHTS

S M T W R F S date week #

TODAY'S GOAL MET	FOOD LOG	calories	fat (g)	protein (g)	carbs (g)	fiber (g)
	Breakfast time:					
MOOD	**Snack** time:					
☹ 2 3 4 ☺	**Lunch** time:					
	Snack time:					
ENERGY LEVEL 🐌 2 3 4 🐇	**Dinner** time:					
	Snack time:					

NUTRIENT TRACKER:

	# of servings	recommended
WATER		8
FRUITS		2-4
VEGETABLES		3-5
GRAINS		6-8
PROTEIN		3-4
DAIRY		2-3
SUGARS	FATS	moderation
VITAMINS/SUPPLEMENTS		

DAILY TOTALS:

calories

carbs   fat

protein   fiber

WORKOUT RATE

great

good

okay

meh

missed

PHYSICAL ACTIVITY	focus	intensity	tin

COMMENTS/THOUGHTS

It is not the challenges we face that make us stronger; it is how we handle them.

START WEIGHT

END WEIGHT

DAYS I TRACKED MY DIET   S   M   T   W   R   F   S

DIET NOTES

THIS WEEK'S MOOD

☹

2

3

4

☺

DAYS I EXERCISED   S   M   T   W   R   F   S

EXERCISE NOTES

THIS WEEK'S ENERGY LEVEL

🐌

2

3

4

🐰

Did I meet this week's goals?

0%   25%   50%   75%   100%

TOTAL WORKOUT TIME

GOALS FOR NEXT WEEK

YOU CAN DO THIS!

S M T W R F S

date

week #

	FOOD LOG	calories	fat (g)	protein (g)	carbs (g)	fiber (g)
TODAY'S GOAL MET	**Breakfast** time:					
MOOD ☹ 2 3 4 ☺	**Snack** time:					
	Lunch time:					
	Snack time:					
ENERGY LEVEL 🐌 2 3 4 🐇	**Dinner** time:					
	Snack time:					

NUTRIENT TRACKER:

	# of servings	recommended
WATER		8
FRUITS		2-4
VEGETABLES		3-5
GRAINS		6-8
PROTEIN		3-4
DAIRY		2-3
SUGARS	FATS	moderation
VITAMINS/SUPPLEMENTS		

DAILY TOTALS:

calories

carbs

fat

protein

fiber

WORKOUT RATE

great

good

okay

meh

missed

PHYSICAL ACTIVITY	focus	intensity	tir

COMMENTS/THOUGHTS

M T W R F S

date

week #

OOD LOG

	calories	fat (g)	protein (g)	carbs (g)	fiber (g)		

eakfast
me:

ack
me:

nch
me:

ack
me:

nner
me:

ack
me:

TODAY'S GOAL MET

MOOD

☹

2

3

4

☺

ENERGY LEVEL

🐌

2

3

4

🐇

NUTRIENT TRACKER:

	# of servings	recommended
WATER		8
FRUITS		2-4
TABLES		3-5
RAINS		6-8
OTEIN		3-4
DAIRY		2-3
JGARS	FATS	moderation
MINS/SUPPLEMENTS		

DAILY TOTALS:

calories

carbs

fat

protein

fiber

WORKOUT RATE

great

good

okay

meh

missed

YSICAL ACTIVITY

	focus	intensity	time

MMENTS/THOUGHTS

S M T W R F S date week

TODAY'S GOAL MET

FOOD LOG

	calories	fat (g)	protein (g)	carbs (g)	fiber (g)
Breakfast time:					
Snack time:					
Lunch time:					
Snack time:					
Dinner time:					
Snack time:					

MOOD

☹
2
3
4
☺

ENERGY LEVEL

🐌
2
3
4
🐇

NUTRIENT TRACKER:

	# of servings	recommended
WATER		8
FRUITS		2-4
VEGETABLES		3-5
GRAINS		6-8
PROTEIN		3-4
DAIRY		2-3
SUGARS	FATS	moderation
VITAMINS/SUPPLEMENTS		

DAILY TOTALS:

calories

carbs   fat

protein   fiber

WORKOUT RATE

great

good

okay

meh

missed

PHYSICAL ACTIVITY

	focus	intensity	ti

COMMENTS/THOUGHTS

S M T W R F S date _____ week # _____

FOOD LOG

	calories	fat (g)	protein (g)	carbs (g)	fiber (g)
Breakfast time:					
Snack time:					
Lunch time:					
Snack time:					
Dinner time:					
Snack time:					

NUTRIENT TRACKER:

	# of servings	recommended
WATER		8
FRUITS		2-4
VEGETABLES		3-5
GRAINS		6-8
PROTEIN		3-4
DAIRY		2-3
SUGARS	FATS	moderation
VITAMINS/SUPPLEMENTS		

DAILY TOTALS:

calories _____

carbs _____   fat _____

protein _____   fiber _____

TODAY'S GOAL MET

MOOD
☹
2
3
4
☺

ENERGY LEVEL
🐌
2
3
4
🐇

WORKOUT RATE
great
good
okay
meh
missed

PHYSICAL ACTIVITY

	focus	intensity	time

COMMENTS/THOUGHTS

S M T W R F S   date _____   week # _____

TODAY'S GOAL MET

MOOD

☹

2

3

4

☺

ENERGY LEVEL

🐌

2

3

4

🐇

WORKOUT RATE

great

good

okay

meh

missed

FOOD LOG	calories	fat (g)	protein (g)	carbs (g)	fiber (g)
Breakfast time:					
Snack time:					
Lunch time:					
Snack time:					
Dinner time:					
Snack time:					

NUTRIENT TRACKER:

	# of servings	recommended
WATER		8
FRUITS		2-4
VEGETABLES		3-5
GRAINS		6-8
PROTEIN		3-4
DAIRY		2-3
SUGARS	FATS	moderation
VITAMINS/SUPPLEMENTS		

DAILY TOTALS:

calories

carbs   fat

protein   fiber

PHYSICAL ACTIVITY	focus	intensity	tim

COMMENTS/THOUGHTS

S M T W R F S   date   week #

FOOD LOG

	calories	fat (g)	protein (g)	carbs (g)	fiber (g)
breakfast time:					
snack time:					
lunch time:					
snack time:					
dinner time:					
snack time:					

TODAY'S GOAL MET

MOOD

☹
2
3
4
☺

ENERGY LEVEL

🐌
2
3
4
🐇

NUTRIENT TRACKER:

	# of servings	recommended
WATER		8
FRUITS		2-4
VEGETABLES		3-5
GRAINS		6-8
PROTEIN		3-4
DAIRY		2-3
SUGARS	FATS	moderation
VITAMINS/SUPPLEMENTS		

DAILY TOTALS:

calories

carbs   fat

protein   fiber

WORKOUT RATE

great

good

okay

meh

missed

PHYSICAL ACTIVITY

	focus	intensity	time

COMMENTS/THOUGHTS

S M T W R F S   date   week

TODAY'S GOAL MET

FOOD LOG

	calories	fat (g)	protein (g)	carbs (g)	fiber (g)
Breakfast time:					
Snack time:					
Lunch time:					
Snack time:					
Dinner time:					
Snack time:					

MOOD

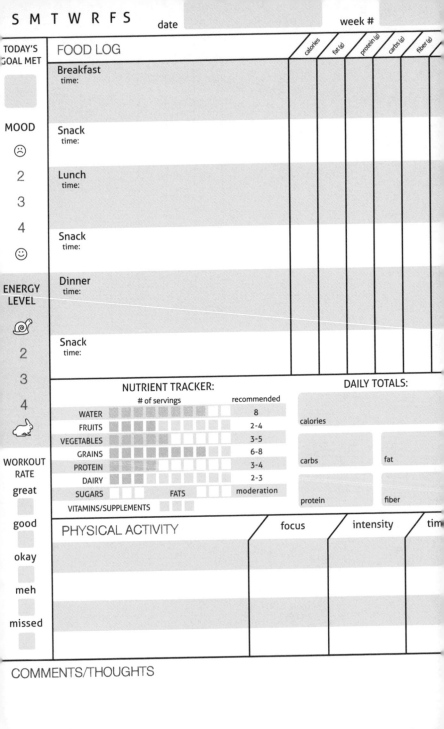

☹
2
3
4
☺

ENERGY LEVEL

🐌
2
3
4
🐇

WORKOUT RATE

great

good

okay

meh

missed

NUTRIENT TRACKER:

	# of servings	recommended
WATER		8
FRUITS		2-4
VEGETABLES		3-5
GRAINS		6-8
PROTEIN		3-4
DAIRY		2-3
SUGARS	FATS	moderation
VITAMINS/SUPPLEMENTS		

DAILY TOTALS:

calories

carbs   fat

protein   fiber

PHYSICAL ACTIVITY

	focus	intensity	tim

COMMENTS/THOUGHTS

> The greater part of our happiness depends on our dispositions and not our circumstances.
>
> -Martha Washington

START WEIGHT

END WEIGHT

DAYS I TRACKED MY DIET S M T W R F S

DIET NOTES

THIS WEEK'S MOOD

☹

2

3

4

☺

DAYS I EXERCISED S M T W R F S

EXERCISE NOTES

THIS WEEK'S ENERGY LEVEL

🐌

2

3

4

🐰

Did I meet this week's goals?

0%   25%   50%   75%   100%

TOTAL WORKOUT TIME

GOALS FOR NEXT WEEK

YOU CAN DO THIS!

S M T W R F S   date _____   week # _____

TODAY'S GOAL MET	FOOD LOG		calories	fat (g)	protein (g)	carbs (g)	fiber (g)
	Breakfast time:						
MOOD ☹	**Snack** time:						
2							
3	**Lunch** time:						
4 ☺	**Snack** time:						
ENERGY LEVEL 🐌	**Dinner** time:						
2	**Snack** time:						

NUTRIENT TRACKER:

	# of servings	recommended
WATER		8
FRUITS		2-4
VEGETABLES		3-5
GRAINS		6-8
PROTEIN		3-4
DAIRY		2-3
SUGARS	FATS	moderation
VITAMINS/SUPPLEMENTS		

DAILY TOTALS:

calories

carbs   fat

protein   fiber

ENERGY LEVEL (continued): 3, 4, 🐰

WORKOUT RATE
- great
- good
- okay
- meh
- missed

PHYSICAL ACTIVITY	focus	intensity	time

COMMENTS/THOUGHTS

M T W R F S

date

week #

OOD LOG

	calories	fat (g)	protein (g)	carbs (g)	fiber (g)		TODAY'S GOAL MET

reakfast
ime:

nack
ime:

unch
me:

nack
me:

inner
me:

nack
me:

TODAY'S GOAL MET

MOOD

☹

2

3

4

☺

ENERGY LEVEL

🐌

2

3

4

🐇

NUTRIENT TRACKER:

	# of servings	recommended
WATER		8
FRUITS		2-4
TABLES		3-5
GRAINS		6-8
PROTEIN		3-4
DAIRY		2-3
SUGARS	FATS	moderation
AMINS/SUPPLEMENTS		

DAILY TOTALS:

calories

carbs

fat

protein

fiber

WORKOUT RATE

great

good

okay

meh

missed

HYSICAL ACTIVITY

	focus	intensity	time

OMMENTS/THOUGHTS

S M T W R F S
date   week #

	FOOD LOG	calories	fat (g)	protein (g)	carbs (g)	fiber (g)
TODAY'S GOAL MET						
	Breakfast time:					
MOOD ☹ 2 3 4 ☺	**Snack** time:					
	Lunch time:					
	Snack time:					
ENERGY LEVEL 🐌 2 3 4 🐇	**Dinner** time:					
	Snack time:					

NUTRIENT TRACKER:

	# of servings	recommended
WATER		8
FRUITS		2-4
VEGETABLES		3-5
GRAINS		6-8
PROTEIN		3-4
DAIRY		2-3
SUGARS	FATS	moderation
VITAMINS/SUPPLEMENTS		

DAILY TOTALS:

calories

carbs   fat

protein   fiber

WORKOUT RATE
great
good
okay
meh
missed

PHYSICAL ACTIVITY	focus	intensity	tim

COMMENTS/THOUGHTS

M T W R F S   date   week #

OOD LOG

	calories	fat (g)	protein (g)	carbs (g)	fiber (g)	
eakfast ne:						
ack ne:						
nch ne:						
ack ne:						
nner ne:						
ack ne:						

NUTRIENT TRACKER:

	# of servings	recommended
WATER		8
FRUITS		2-4
ABLES		3-5
RAINS		6-8
OTEIN		3-4
DAIRY		2-3
UGARS	FATS	moderation
MINS/SUPPLEMENTS		

DAILY TOTALS:

calories

carbs   fat

protein   fiber

YSICAL ACTIVITY

	focus	intensity	time

MMENTS/THOUGHTS

TODAY'S GOAL MET

MOOD

☹
2
3
4
☺

ENERGY LEVEL

🐌
2
3
4
🐇

WORKOUT RATE

great

good

okay

meh

missed

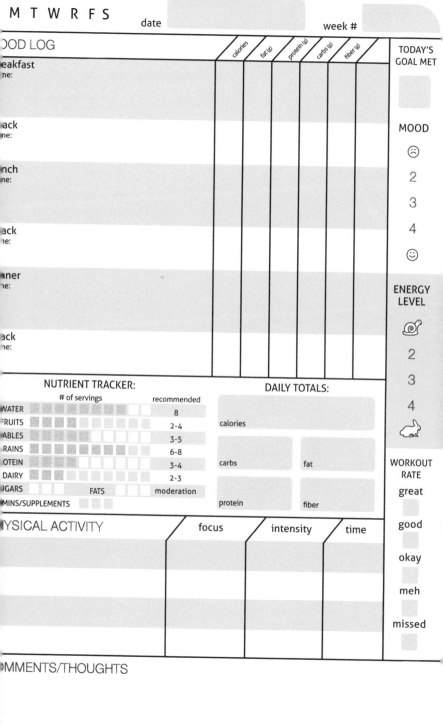

S M T W R F S

date   week #

TODAY'S GOAL MET	FOOD LOG	calories	fat (g)	protein (g)	carbs (g)	fiber (g)
	Breakfast time:					
MOOD ☹ 2 3 4 ☺	**Snack** time:					
	Lunch time:					
	Snack time:					
ENERGY LEVEL 🐌 2 3 4 🐇	**Dinner** time:					
	Snack time:					

NUTRIENT TRACKER:

	# of servings	recommended
WATER		8
FRUITS		2-4
VEGETABLES		3-5
GRAINS		6-8
PROTEIN		3-4
DAIRY		2-3
SUGARS	FATS	moderation
VITAMINS/SUPPLEMENTS		

DAILY TOTALS:

calories

carbs   fat

protein   fiber

WORKOUT RATE

great

good

okay

meh

missed

PHYSICAL ACTIVITY	focus	intensity	ti

COMMENTS/THOUGHTS

M T W R F S   date _____   week # ____

FOOD LOG

		calories	fat (g)	protein (g)	carbs (g)	fiber (g)	
Breakfast time:							
Snack time:							
Lunch time:							
Snack time:							
Dinner time:							
Snack time:							

TODAY'S GOAL MET

MOOD
- ☹
- 2
- 3
- 4
- ☺

ENERGY LEVEL
- 🐌
- 2
- 3
- 4
- 🐇

WORKOUT RATE
- great
- good
- okay
- meh
- missed

NUTRIENT TRACKER:

	# of servings	recommended
WATER		8
FRUITS		2-4
VEGETABLES		3-5
GRAINS		6-8
PROTEIN		3-4
DAIRY		2-3
SUGARS	FATS	moderation
VITAMINS/SUPPLEMENTS		

DAILY TOTALS:

calories

carbs   fat

protein   fiber

PHYSICAL ACTIVITY

	focus	intensity	time

COMMENTS/THOUGHTS

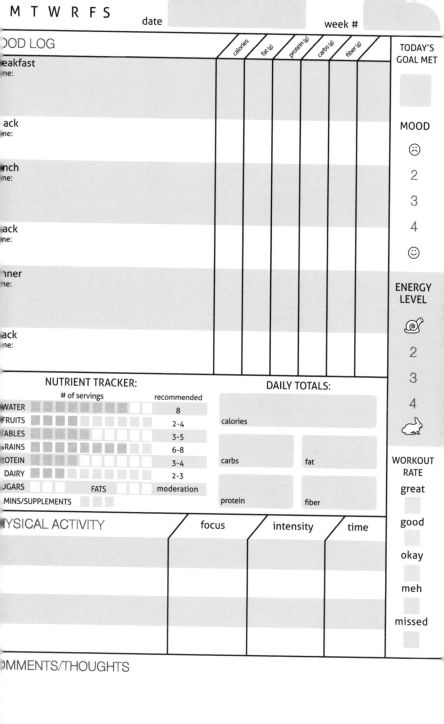

S M T W R F S   date   week #

FOOD LOG	calories	fat (g)	protein (g)	carbs (g)	fiber (g)
Breakfast time:					
Snack time:					
Lunch time:					
Snack time:					
Dinner time:					
Snack time:					

TODAY'S GOAL MET

MOOD

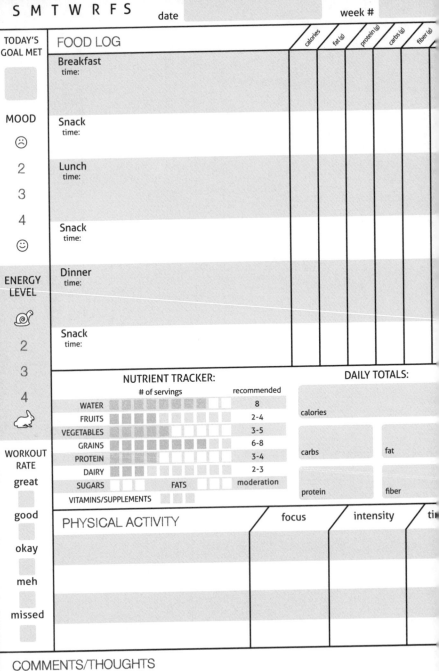

2

3

4

☺

ENERGY LEVEL

🐌

2

3

4

🐇

WORKOUT RATE

great

good

okay

meh

missed

NUTRIENT TRACKER:

	# of servings	recommended
WATER		8
FRUITS		2-4
VEGETABLES		3-5
GRAINS		6-8
PROTEIN		3-4
DAIRY		2-3
SUGARS	FATS	moderation
VITAMINS/SUPPLEMENTS		

DAILY TOTALS:

calories

carbs   fat

protein   fiber

PHYSICAL ACTIVITY	focus	intensity	ti

COMMENTS/THOUGHTS

date   week #

Have faith in yourself.
It is the key to success.

START WEIGHT

END WEIGHT

AYS I TRACKED MY DIET   S   M   T   W   R   F   S

ET NOTES

THIS WEEK'S MOOD

☹

2

3

4

☺

YS I EXERCISED   S   M   T   W   R   F   S

ERCISE NOTES

THIS WEEK'S ENERGY LEVEL

🐌

2

3

4

🐇

Did I meet this week's goals?

0%   25%   50%   75%   100%

TOTAL WORKOUT TIME

OALS FOR NEXT WEEK

S M T W R F S date week #

	FOOD LOG	calories	fat (g)	protein (g)	carbs (g)	fiber (g)
TODAY'S GOAL MET	**Breakfast** time:					
MOOD ☹ 2 3 4 ☺	**Snack** time:					
	Lunch time:					
	Snack time:					
ENERGY LEVEL 🐌 2 3 4 🐇	**Dinner** time:					
	Snack time:					

NUTRIENT TRACKER:

	# of servings	recommended
WATER		8
FRUITS		2-4
VEGETABLES		3-5
GRAINS		6-8
PROTEIN		3-4
DAIRY		2-3
SUGARS	FATS	moderation
VITAMINS/SUPPLEMENTS		

DAILY TOTALS:

calories

carbs   fat

protein   fiber

WORKOUT RATE
great
good
okay
meh
missed

PHYSICAL ACTIVITY	focus	intensity	tir

COMMENTS/THOUGHTS

M T W R F S   date   week #

OOD LOG

	calories	fat (g)	protein (g)	carbs (g)	fiber (g)
eakfast me:					
ack me:					
nch ne:					
ack me:					
nner ne:					
ack me:					

TODAY'S GOAL MET

MOOD

☹

2

3

4

☺

ENERGY LEVEL

🐌

2

3

4

🐰

NUTRIENT TRACKER:

	# of servings	recommended
WATER		8
FRUITS		2-4
ABLES		3-5
RAINS		6-8
ROTEIN		3-4
DAIRY		2-3
JGARS	FATS	moderation
MINS/SUPPLEMENTS		

DAILY TOTALS:

calories

carbs   fat

protein   fiber

WORKOUT RATE

great

good

okay

meh

missed

HYSICAL ACTIVITY

	focus	intensity	time

MMENTS/THOUGHTS

S M T W R F S   date ____   week # ____

	FOOD LOG	calories	fat (g)	protein (g)	carbs (g)	fiber (g)
TODAY'S GOAL MET	**Breakfast** time:					
MOOD ☹ 2 3 4 ☺	**Snack** time:					
	Lunch time:					
	Snack time:					
ENERGY LEVEL 🐌 2 3 4 🐇	**Dinner** time:					
	Snack time:					

NUTRIENT TRACKER:

	# of servings	recommended
WATER		8
FRUITS		2-4
VEGETABLES		3-5
GRAINS		6-8
PROTEIN		3-4
DAIRY		2-3
SUGARS	FATS	moderation
VITAMINS/SUPPLEMENTS		

DAILY TOTALS:

calories

carbs   fat

protein   fiber

WORKOUT RATE
great
good
okay
meh
missed

PHYSICAL ACTIVITY	focus	intensity	ti

COMMENTS/THOUGHTS

M T W R F S   date   week #

FOOD LOG

	calories	fat (g)	protein (g)	carbs (g)	fiber (g)
Breakfast time:					
Snack time:					
Lunch time:					
Snack time:					
Dinner time:					
Snack time:					

TODAY'S GOAL MET

MOOD

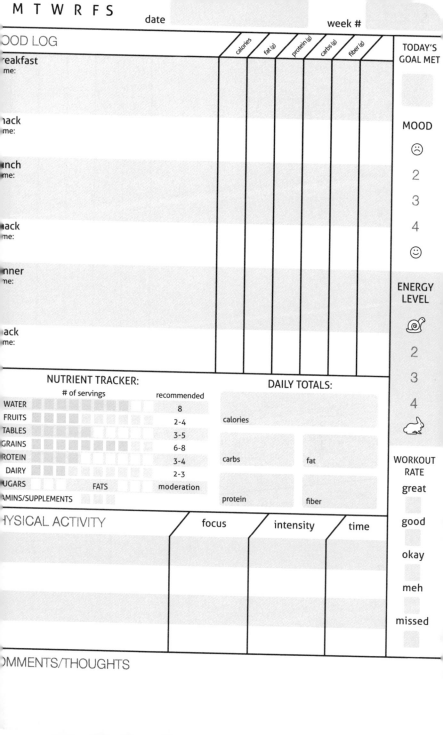
2
3
4
☺

ENERGY LEVEL

🐌
2
3
4
🐇

WORKOUT RATE

great

good

okay

meh

missed

NUTRIENT TRACKER:

	# of servings	recommended
WATER		8
FRUITS		2-4
VEGETABLES		3-5
GRAINS		6-8
PROTEIN		3-4
DAIRY		2-3
SUGARS	FATS	moderation
VITAMINS/SUPPLEMENTS		

DAILY TOTALS:

calories

carbs   fat

protein   fiber

PHYSICAL ACTIVITY

	focus	intensity	time

COMMENTS/THOUGHTS

S M T W R F S   date   week

TODAY'S GOAL MET

FOOD LOG

	calories	fat (g)	protein (g)	carbs (g)	fiber (g)
Breakfast time:					
Snack time:					
Lunch time:					
Snack time:					
Dinner time:					
Snack time:					

MOOD

☹

2

3

4

☺

ENERGY LEVEL

🐌

2

3

4

🐇

NUTRIENT TRACKER:

	# of servings	recommended
WATER		8
FRUITS		2-4
VEGETABLES		3-5
GRAINS		6-8
PROTEIN		3-4
DAIRY		2-3
SUGARS	FATS	moderation
VITAMINS/SUPPLEMENTS		

DAILY TOTALS:

calories

carbs

fat

protein

fiber

WORKOUT RATE

great

good

okay

meh

missed

PHYSICAL ACTIVITY

	focus	intensity	tir

COMMENTS/THOUGHTS

M T W R F S

date _____   week # _____

FOOD LOG

	calories	fat (g)	protein (g)	carbs (g)	fiber (g)
Breakfast time:					
Snack time:					
Lunch time:					
Snack time:					
Dinner time:					
Snack time:					

TODAY'S GOAL MET

MOOD

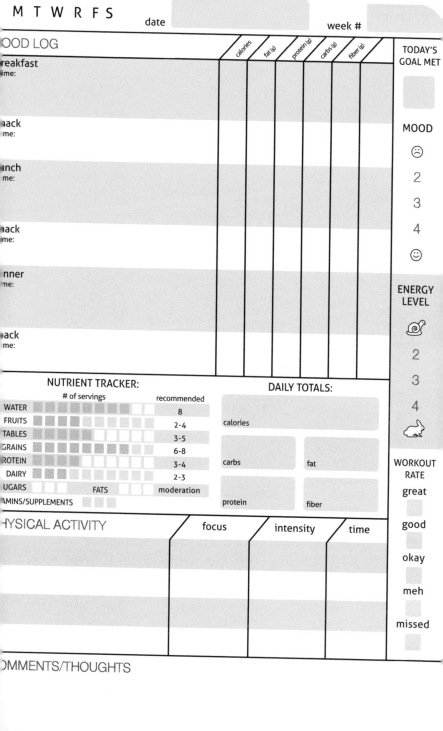

☹
2
3
4
☺

ENERGY LEVEL

🐌
2
3
4
🐇

NUTRIENT TRACKER:

	# of servings	recommended
WATER		8
FRUITS		2-4
VEGETABLES		3-5
GRAINS		6-8
PROTEIN		3-4
DAIRY		2-3
SUGARS	FATS	moderation
VITAMINS/SUPPLEMENTS		

DAILY TOTALS:

calories

carbs   fat

protein   fiber

WORKOUT RATE

great
good
okay
meh
missed

PHYSICAL ACTIVITY

	focus	intensity	time

COMMENTS/THOUGHTS

S M T W R F S date   week

TODAY'S GOAL MET	FOOD LOG	calories	fat (g)	protein (g)	carbs (g)	fiber (g)
	Breakfast time:					
MOOD ☹ 2 3 4 ☺	**Snack** time:					
	Lunch time:					
	Snack time:					
ENERGY LEVEL 🐌 2 3 4 🐇	**Dinner** time:					
	Snack time:					

NUTRIENT TRACKER:

	# of servings	recommended
WATER		8
FRUITS		2-4
VEGETABLES		3-5
GRAINS		6-8
PROTEIN		3-4
DAIRY		2-3
SUGARS	FATS	moderation
VITAMINS/SUPPLEMENTS		

DAILY TOTALS:

calories

carbs   fat

protein   fiber

WORKOUT RATE	PHYSICAL ACTIVITY	focus	intensity	tir
great				
good				
okay				
meh				
missed				

COMMENTS/THOUGHTS

> Greatness lies not in being strong,
> but in the right use of strength.
>
> -Henry Ward Beecher

START WEIGHT

END WEIGHT

DAYS I TRACKED MY DIET   S   M   T   W   R   F   S

DIET NOTES

THIS WEEK'S MOOD

☹

2

3

4

☺

DAYS I EXERCISED   S   M   T   W   R   F   S

EXERCISE NOTES

THIS WEEK'S ENERGY LEVEL

🐌

2

3

4

🐇

Did I meet this week's goals?

0%   25%   50%   75%   100%

TOTAL WORKOUT TIME

GOALS FOR NEXT WEEK

YOU CAN DO THIS!

S M T W R F S   date ____   week # ____

	FOOD LOG	calories	fat (g)	protein (g)	carbs (g)	fiber (g)
TODAY'S GOAL MET	**Breakfast** time:					
	Snack time:					
MOOD ☹ 2 3 4 ☺	**Lunch** time:					
	Snack time:					
ENERGY LEVEL 🐌 2 3 4 🐰	**Dinner** time:					
	Snack time:					

NUTRIENT TRACKER:

	# of servings	recommended
WATER		8
FRUITS		2-4
VEGETABLES		3-5
GRAINS		6-8
PROTEIN		3-4
DAIRY		2-3
SUGARS	FATS	moderation
VITAMINS/SUPPLEMENTS		

DAILY TOTALS:

calories

carbs   fat

protein   fiber

WORKOUT RATE great good okay meh missed	PHYSICAL ACTIVITY	focus	intensity	tim

COMMENTS/THOUGHTS

M T W R F S

date   week #

FOOD LOG

	calories	fat (g)	protein (g)	carbs (g)	fiber (g)	

Breakfast
Time:

Snack
Time:

Lunch
Time:

Snack
Time:

Dinner
Time:

Snack
Time:

NUTRIENT TRACKER:

	# of servings	recommended
WATER		8
FRUITS		2-4
VEGETABLES		3-5
GRAINS		6-8
PROTEIN		3-4
DAIRY		2-3
SUGARS	FATS	moderation
VITAMINS/SUPPLEMENTS		

DAILY TOTALS:

calories

carbs   fat

protein   fiber

PHYSICAL ACTIVITY

	focus	intensity	time

COMMENTS/THOUGHTS

TODAY'S GOAL MET

MOOD
☹
2
3
4
☺

ENERGY LEVEL
🐌
2
3
4
🐰

WORKOUT RATE
great

good

okay

meh

missed

S M T W R F S   date   week #

	FOOD LOG	calories	fat (g)	protein (g)	carbs (g)	fiber (g)
TODAY'S GOAL MET	**Breakfast** time:					
MOOD ☹ 2 3 4 ☺	**Snack** time:					
	Lunch time:					
	Snack time:					
ENERGY LEVEL 🐌 2 3 4 🐰	**Dinner** time:					
	Snack time:					

NUTRIENT TRACKER:

DAILY TOTALS:

	# of servings	recommended
WATER		8
FRUITS		2-4
VEGETABLES		3-5
GRAINS		6-8
PROTEIN		3-4
DAIRY		2-3
SUGARS	FATS	moderation
VITAMINS/SUPPLEMENTS		

calories

carbs   fat

protein   fiber

WORKOUT RATE
great
good
okay
meh
missed

PHYSICAL ACTIVITY	focus	intensity	tir

COMMENTS/THOUGHTS

M T W R F S

date   week #

FOOD LOG

	calories	fat (g)	protein (g)	carbs (g)	fiber (g)
breakfast time:					
snack time:					
lunch time:					
snack time:					
dinner time:					
snack time:					

TODAY'S GOAL MET

MOOD

☹

2

3

4

☺

ENERGY LEVEL

🐌

2

3

4

🐇

NUTRIENT TRACKER:

	# of servings	recommended
WATER		8
FRUITS		2-4
VEGETABLES		3-5
GRAINS		6-8
PROTEIN		3-4
DAIRY		2-3
SUGARS	FATS	moderation
VITAMINS/SUPPLEMENTS		

DAILY TOTALS:

calories

carbs   fat

protein   fiber

WORKOUT RATE

great

good

okay

meh

missed

PHYSICAL ACTIVITY

	focus	intensity	time

COMMENTS/THOUGHTS

S M T W R F S   date _____   week # _____

TODAY'S GOAL MET	FOOD LOG	calories	fat (g)	protein (g)	carbs (g)	fiber (g)
	Breakfast time:					
MOOD ☹ 2 3 4 ☺	**Snack** time:					
	Lunch time:					
	Snack time:					
ENERGY LEVEL 🐌 2 3 4 🐇	**Dinner** time:					
	Snack time:					

NUTRIENT TRACKER:

	# of servings	recommended
WATER		8
FRUITS		2-4
VEGETABLES		3-5
GRAINS		6-8
PROTEIN		3-4
DAIRY		2-3
SUGARS	FATS	moderation
VITAMINS/SUPPLEMENTS		

DAILY TOTALS:

calories

carbs   fat

protein   fiber

WORKOUT RATE
great
good
okay
meh
missed

PHYSICAL ACTIVITY	focus	intensity	time

COMMENTS/THOUGHTS

M T W R F S

date   week #

OOD LOG

	calories	fat (g)	protein (g)	carbs (g)	fiber (g)
eakfast me:					
ack me:					
nch me:					
ack me:					
nner me:					
ack me:					

TODAY'S GOAL MET

MOOD

☹
2
3
4
☺

ENERGY LEVEL

🐌
2
3
4
🐇

NUTRIENT TRACKER:

	# of servings	recommended
WATER		8
FRUITS		2-4
TABLES		3-5
GRAINS		6-8
ROTEIN		3-4
DAIRY		2-3
UGARS	FATS	moderation
MINS/SUPPLEMENTS		

DAILY TOTALS:

calories

carbs   fat

protein   fiber

WORKOUT RATE

great

good

okay

meh

missed

HYSICAL ACTIVITY

	focus	intensity	time

OMMENTS/THOUGHTS

S M T W R F S date week

TODAY'S GOAL MET

FOOD LOG

	calories	fat (g)	protein (g)	carbs (g)	fiber (g)
Breakfast time:					
Snack time:					
Lunch time:					
Snack time:					
Dinner time:					
Snack time:					

MOOD

☹
2
3
4
☺

ENERGY LEVEL

🐌
2
3
4
🐇

WORKOUT RATE

great
good
okay
meh
missed

NUTRIENT TRACKER:

	# of servings	recommended
WATER		8
FRUITS		2-4
VEGETABLES		3-5
GRAINS		6-8
PROTEIN		3-4
DAIRY		2-3
SUGARS	FATS	moderation
VITAMINS/SUPPLEMENTS		

DAILY TOTALS:

calories

carbs   fat

protein   fiber

PHYSICAL ACTIVITY

	focus	intensity	ti

COMMENTS/THOUGHTS

> Never forget that even the tiniest effort,
> if it is well intentioned and well thought out,
> can make a world of difference.

DAYS I TRACKED MY DIET S M T W R F S	**START WEIGHT**
DIET NOTES	
	END WEIGHT
	THIS WEEK'S MOOD ☹ 2 3 4 ☺
DAYS I EXERCISED S M T W R F S	
EXERCISE NOTES	**THIS WEEK'S ENERGY LEVEL** 🐌 2 3 4 🐇
Did I meet this week's goals? 0% 25% 50% 75% 100%	**TOTAL WORKOUT TIME**

GOALS FOR NEXT WEEK

YOU CAN DO THIS!

S M T W R F S   date   week #

TODAY'S GOAL MET	FOOD LOG	calories	fat (g)	protein (g)	carbs (g)	fiber (g)
	Breakfast time:					
MOOD	**Snack** time:					
☹						
2	**Lunch** time:					
3						
4						
☺	**Snack** time:					
ENERGY LEVEL	**Dinner** time:					
🐌						
2	**Snack** time:					

NUTRIENT TRACKER:

# of servings   recommended

	# of servings	recommended
WATER		8
FRUITS		2-4
VEGETABLES		3-5
GRAINS		6-8
PROTEIN		3-4
DAIRY		2-3
SUGARS	FATS	moderation
VITAMINS/SUPPLEMENTS		

DAILY TOTALS:

calories

carbs   fat

protein   fiber

WORKOUT RATE

great

good

okay

meh

missed

PHYSICAL ACTIVITY	focus	intensity	tir

COMMENTS/THOUGHTS

M T W R F S

date _____   week # _____

FOOD LOG

	calories	fat (g)	protein (g)	carbs (g)	fiber (g)
Breakfast time:					
Snack time:					
Lunch time:					
Snack time:					
Dinner time:					
Snack time:					

NUTRIENT TRACKER:

	# of servings	recommended
WATER		8
FRUITS		2-4
VEGETABLES		3-5
GRAINS		6-8
PROTEIN		3-4
DAIRY		2-3
SUGARS	FATS	moderation
VITAMINS/SUPPLEMENTS		

DAILY TOTALS:

calories _____

carbs _____   fat _____

protein _____   fiber _____

PHYSICAL ACTIVITY

	focus	intensity	time

TODAY'S GOAL MET

MOOD

☹
2
3
4
☺

ENERGY LEVEL

🐌
2
3
4
🐇

WORKOUT RATE

great
good
okay
meh
missed

COMMENTS/THOUGHTS

S M T W R F S   date _____   week # _____

	FOOD LOG	calories	fat (g)	protein (g)	carbs (g)	fiber (g)
TODAY'S GOAL MET	**Breakfast** time:					
MOOD ☹ 2 3 4 ☺	**Snack** time:					
	Lunch time:					
ENERGY LEVEL 🐌 2 3 4 🐇	**Snack** time:					
	Dinner time:					
	Snack time:					

NUTRIENT TRACKER:

	# of servings	recommended
WATER		8
FRUITS		2-4
VEGETABLES		3-5
GRAINS		6-8
PROTEIN		3-4
DAIRY		2-3
SUGARS	FATS	moderation
VITAMINS/SUPPLEMENTS		

DAILY TOTALS:

calories

carbs   fat

protein   fiber

WORKOUT RATE
great
good
okay
meh
missed

PHYSICAL ACTIVITY	focus	intensity	ti

COMMENTS/THOUGHTS

M T W R F S   date   week #

~OOD LOG

	calories	fat (g)	protein (g)	carbs (g)	fiber (g)
~reakfast ~ime:					
~nack ~me:					
~unch ~me:					
~ack ~me:					
~inner ~me:					
~ack ~me:					

TODAY'S GOAL MET

MOOD

☹

2

3

4

☺

ENERGY LEVEL

🐌

2

3

4

🐇

NUTRIENT TRACKER:

	# of servings	recommended
WATER		8
FRUITS		2-4
~TABLES		3-5
~GRAINS		6-8
~ROTEIN		3-4
DAIRY		2-3
~UGARS	FATS	moderation
~AMINS/SUPPLEMENTS		

DAILY TOTALS:

calories

carbs   fat

protein   fiber

WORKOUT RATE

great

good

okay

meh

missed

~HYSICAL ACTIVITY

	focus	intensity	time

~OMMENTS/THOUGHTS

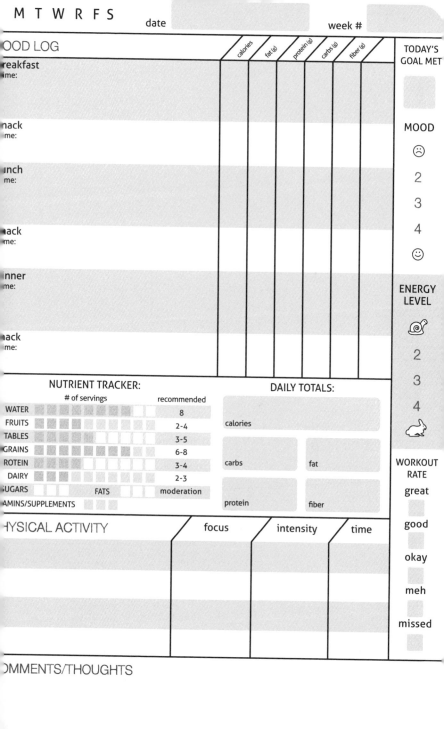

S M T W R F S

date

week #

	FOOD LOG	calories	fat (g)	protein (g)	carbs (g)	fiber (g)
TODAY'S GOAL MET	**Breakfast** time:					
MOOD ☹ 2 3 4 ☺	**Snack** time:					
	Lunch time:					
	Snack time:					
ENERGY LEVEL 🐌 2 3 4 🐇	**Dinner** time:					
	Snack time:					

NUTRIENT TRACKER:

	# of servings	recommended
WATER		8
FRUITS		2-4
VEGETABLES		3-5
GRAINS		6-8
PROTEIN		3-4
DAIRY		2-3
SUGARS	FATS	moderation
VITAMINS/SUPPLEMENTS		

DAILY TOTALS:

calories

carbs   fat

protein   fiber

WORKOUT RATE

great

good

okay

meh

missed

PHYSICAL ACTIVITY	focus	intensity	tim

COMMENTS/THOUGHTS

M T W R F S   date [ ]   week #

FOOD LOG

	calories	fat (g)	protein (g)	carbs (g)	fiber (g)	
breakfast time:						
snack time:						
lunch time:						
snack time:						
dinner time:						
snack time:						

TODAY'S GOAL MET

[ ]

MOOD

☹
2
3
4
☺

ENERGY LEVEL

🐌
2
3
4
🐇

WORKOUT RATE

great [ ]
good [ ]
okay [ ]
meh [ ]
missed [ ]

NUTRIENT TRACKER:

	# of servings	recommended
WATER		8
FRUITS		2-4
VEGETABLES		3-5
GRAINS		6-8
PROTEIN		3-4
DAIRY		2-3
SUGARS	FATS	moderation
VITAMINS/SUPPLEMENTS		

DAILY TOTALS:

calories

carbs	fat

protein	fiber

PHYSICAL ACTIVITY

	focus	intensity	time

COMMENTS/THOUGHTS

S M T W R F S   date _____   week # _____

TODAY'S GOAL MET	FOOD LOG	calories	fat (g)	protein (g)	carbs (g)	fiber (g)
	Breakfast time:					
	Snack time:					
MOOD	**Lunch** time:					
☹						
2						
3	**Snack** time:					
4						
☺						
ENERGY LEVEL	**Dinner** time:					
🐌						
2	**Snack** time:					
3						

NUTRIENT TRACKER:

	# of servings	recommended
WATER		8
FRUITS		2-4
VEGETABLES		3-5
GRAINS		6-8
PROTEIN		3-4
DAIRY		2-3
SUGARS	FATS	moderation
VITAMINS/SUPPLEMENTS		

DAILY TOTALS:

calories

carbs   fat

protein   fiber

ENERGY LEVEL

🐌

2

3

4

🐰

WORKOUT RATE

great

good

okay

meh

missed

PHYSICAL ACTIVITY	focus	intensity	time

COMMENTS/THOUGHTS

The difference between a dream and a reality
is the action we take in between.

START WEIGHT

END WEIGHT

DAYS I TRACKED MY DIET   S   M   T   W   R   F   S

DIET NOTES

THIS WEEK'S MOOD

☹

2

3

4

☺

DAYS I EXERCISED   S   M   T   W   R   F   S

EXERCISE NOTES

THIS WEEK'S ENERGY LEVEL

🐌

2

3

4

🐰

Did I meet this week's goals?

0%   25%   50%   75%   100%

TOTAL WORKOUT TIME

GOALS FOR NEXT WEEK

YOU CAN DO THIS!

S M T W R F S   date   week #

TODAY'S GOAL MET	FOOD LOG	calories	fat (g)	protein (g)	carbs (g)	fiber (g)
	Breakfast time:					
MOOD ☹ 2 3 4 ☺	**Snack** time:					
	Lunch time:					
	Snack time:					
ENERGY LEVEL 🐌 2 3 4 🐇	**Dinner** time:					
	Snack time:					

NUTRIENT TRACKER:

	# of servings	recommended
WATER		8
FRUITS		2-4
VEGETABLES		3-5
GRAINS		6-8
PROTEIN		3-4
DAIRY		2-3
SUGARS	FATS	moderation
VITAMINS/SUPPLEMENTS		

DAILY TOTALS:

calories

carbs   fat

protein   fiber

WORKOUT RATE

great

good

okay

meh

missed

PHYSICAL ACTIVITY	focus	intensity	tim

COMMENTS/THOUGHTS

S M T W R F S   date [ ]   week # [ ]

FOOD LOG

	calories	fat (g)	protein (g)	carbs (g)	fiber (g)
Breakfast time:					
Snack time:					
Lunch time:					
Snack time:					
Dinner time:					
Snack time:					

TODAY'S GOAL MET

MOOD
☹
2
3
4
☺

ENERGY LEVEL
🐌
2
3
4
🐇

WORKOUT RATE
great
good
okay
meh
missed

NUTRIENT TRACKER:

	# of servings	recommended
WATER		8
FRUITS		2-4
ETABLES		3-5
GRAINS		6-8
PROTEIN		3-4
DAIRY		2-3
SUGARS	FATS	moderation
AMINS/SUPPLEMENTS		

DAILY TOTALS:

calories

carbs   fat

protein   fiber

HYSICAL ACTIVITY

	focus	intensity	time

OMMENTS/THOUGHTS

S M T W R F S   date   week

TODAY'S GOAL MET

FOOD LOG

	calories	fat (g)	protein (g)	carbs (g)	fiber (g)
Breakfast time:					
Snack time:					
Lunch time:					
Snack time:					
Dinner time:					
Snack time:					

MOOD

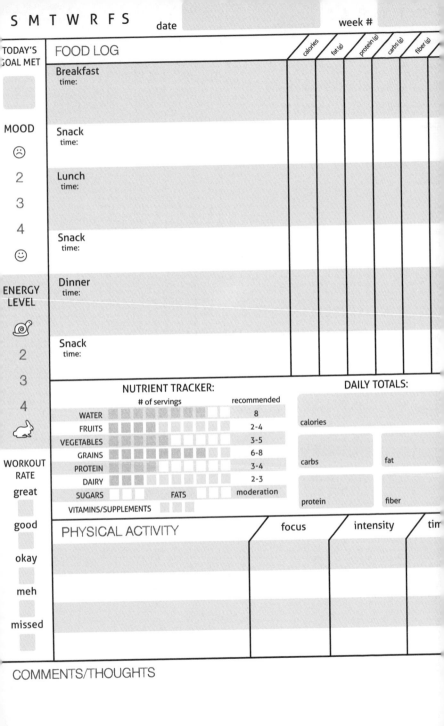

☹
2
3
4
☺

ENERGY LEVEL

🐌
2
3
4
🐇

NUTRIENT TRACKER:

	# of servings	recommended
WATER		8
FRUITS		2-4
VEGETABLES		3-5
GRAINS		6-8
PROTEIN		3-4
DAIRY		2-3
SUGARS	FATS	moderation
VITAMINS/SUPPLEMENTS		

DAILY TOTALS:

calories

carbs   fat

protein   fiber

WORKOUT RATE

great

good

okay

meh

missed

PHYSICAL ACTIVITY

	focus	intensity	tim

COMMENTS/THOUGHTS

M T W R F S   date _____   week # _____

FOOD LOG

	calories	fat (g)	protein (g)	carbs (g)	fiber (g)	
Breakfast time:						
Snack time:						
Lunch time:						
Snack time:						
Dinner time:						
Snack time:						

TODAY'S GOAL MET

MOOD
☹
2
3
4
☺

ENERGY LEVEL
🐌
2
3
4
🐇

NUTRIENT TRACKER:

	# of servings	recommended
WATER		8
FRUITS		2-4
VEGETABLES		3-5
GRAINS		6-8
PROTEIN		3-4
DAIRY		2-3
SUGARS	FATS	moderation
VITAMINS/SUPPLEMENTS		

DAILY TOTALS:

calories

carbs   fat

protein   fiber

WORKOUT RATE
great
good
okay
meh
missed

PHYSICAL ACTIVITY

	focus	intensity	time

COMMENTS/THOUGHTS

S M T W R F S   date   week

TODAY'S GOAL MET	FOOD LOG	calories	fat (g)	protein (g)	carbs (g)	fiber (g)
	Breakfast time:					
MOOD ☹ 2 3 4 ☺	**Snack** time:					
	Lunch time:					
	Snack time:					
ENERGY LEVEL 🐌 2 3 4 🐇	**Dinner** time:					
	Snack time:					

NUTRIENT TRACKER:

	# of servings	recommended
WATER		8
FRUITS		2-4
VEGETABLES		3-5
GRAINS		6-8
PROTEIN		3-4
DAIRY		2-3
SUGARS	FATS	moderation
VITAMINS/SUPPLEMENTS		

DAILY TOTALS:

calories

carbs   fat

protein   fiber

WORKOUT RATE

great
good
okay
meh
missed

PHYSICAL ACTIVITY	focus	intensity	tim

COMMENTS/THOUGHTS

M T W R F S   date   week #

OOD LOG

	calories	fat (g)	protein (g)	carbs (g)	fiber (g)
reakfast me:					
ack me:					
nch ne:					
ack ne:					
nner me:					
ack me:					

TODAY'S GOAL MET

MOOD

☹

2

3

4

☺

ENERGY LEVEL

🐌

2

3

4

🐇

NUTRIENT TRACKER:

	# of servings	recommended
WATER		8
FRUITS		2-4
TABLES		3-5
GRAINS		6-8
ROTEIN		3-4
DAIRY		2-3
UGARS	FATS	moderation
MINS/SUPPLEMENTS		

DAILY TOTALS:

calories

carbs   fat

protein   fiber

WORKOUT RATE

great

good

okay

meh

missed

HYSICAL ACTIVITY

	focus	intensity	time

OMMENTS/THOUGHTS

S M T W R F S   date   week #

TODAY'S GOAL MET	FOOD LOG	calories	fat (g)	protein (g)	carbs (g)	fiber (g)
	Breakfast time:					
MOOD ☹ 2 3 4 ☺	**Snack** time:					
	Lunch time:					
	Snack time:					
ENERGY LEVEL 🐌 2 3 4 🐇	**Dinner** time:					
	Snack time:					

NUTRIENT TRACKER:

# of servings — recommended

		recommended
WATER		8
FRUITS		2-4
VEGETABLES		3-5
GRAINS		6-8
PROTEIN		3-4
DAIRY		2-3
SUGARS	FATS	moderation
VITAMINS/SUPPLEMENTS		

DAILY TOTALS:

calories

carbs   fat

protein   fiber

WORKOUT RATE
great
good
okay
meh
missed

PHYSICAL ACTIVITY	focus	intensity	ti

COMMENTS/THOUGHTS

START WEIGHT

END WEIGHT

> Do what you can,
> with what you have, where you are.
> -Theodore Roosevelt

DAYS I TRACKED MY DIET   S   M   T   W   R   F   S

DIET NOTES

THIS WEEK'S MOOD

☹

2

3

4

☺

DAYS I EXERCISED   S   M   T   W   R   F   S

EXERCISE NOTES

THIS WEEK'S ENERGY LEVEL

🐌

2

3

4

🐇

Did I meet this week's goals?

0%   25%   50%   75%   100%

TOTAL WORKOUT TIME

GOALS FOR NEXT WEEK

YOU CAN DO THIS!

S M T W R F S

date

week #

TODAY'S GOAL MET	FOOD LOG		calories	fat (g)	protein (g)	carbs (g)	fiber (g)
	Breakfast time:						
MOOD ☹ 2 3 4 ☺	**Snack** time:						
	Lunch time:						
	Snack time:						
ENERGY LEVEL 🐌 2 3 4 🐇	**Dinner** time:						
	Snack time:						

NUTRIENT TRACKER:

	# of servings	recommended
WATER		8
FRUITS		2-4
VEGETABLES		3-5
GRAINS		6-8
PROTEIN		3-4
DAIRY		2-3
SUGARS	FATS	moderation
VITAMINS/SUPPLEMENTS		

DAILY TOTALS:

calories

carbs   fat

protein   fiber

WORKOUT RATE

great

good

okay

meh

missed

PHYSICAL ACTIVITY	focus	intensity	tim

COMMENTS/THOUGHTS

M T W R F S

date   week #

FOOD LOG

	calories	fat (g)	protein (g)	carbs (g)	fiber (g)
Breakfast time:					
Snack time:					
Lunch time:					
Snack time:					
Dinner time:					
Snack time:					

TODAY'S GOAL MET

MOOD

☹
2
3
4
☺

ENERGY LEVEL

🐌
2
3
4
🐇

WORKOUT RATE

great
good
okay
meh
missed

NUTRIENT TRACKER:

	# of servings	recommended
WATER		8
FRUITS		2-4
VEGETABLES		3-5
GRAINS		6-8
PROTEIN		3-4
DAIRY		2-3
SUGARS	FATS	moderation
VITAMINS/SUPPLEMENTS		

DAILY TOTALS:

calories

carbs

fat

protein

fiber

PHYSICAL ACTIVITY

	focus	intensity	time

COMMENTS/THOUGHTS

S M T W R F S   date   week #

	FOOD LOG	calories	fat (g)	protein (g)	carbs (g)	fiber (g)
TODAY'S GOAL MET						
	Breakfast time:					
MOOD	**Snack** time:					
☹ 2 3 4 ☺	**Lunch** time:					
	Snack time:					
ENERGY LEVEL	**Dinner** time:					
🐌 2 3 4 🐇	**Snack** time:					

NUTRIENT TRACKER:

	# of servings	recommended
WATER		8
FRUITS		2-4
VEGETABLES		3-5
GRAINS		6-8
PROTEIN		3-4
DAIRY		2-3
SUGARS	FATS	moderation
VITAMINS/SUPPLEMENTS		

DAILY TOTALS:

calories

carbs   fat

protein   fiber

WORKOUT RATE

great

good

okay

meh

missed

PHYSICAL ACTIVITY	focus	intensity	time

COMMENTS/THOUGHTS

M T W R F S   date   week #

FOOD LOG

	calories	fat (g)	protein (g)	carbs (g)	fiber (g)	
Breakfast time:						
Snack time:						
Lunch time:						
Snack time:						
Dinner time:						
Snack time:						

TODAY'S GOAL MET

MOOD

☹

2

3

4

☺

ENERGY LEVEL

🐌

2

3

4

🐇

WORKOUT RATE

great

good

okay

meh

missed

NUTRIENT TRACKER:

	# of servings	recommended
WATER		8
FRUITS		2-4
VEGETABLES		3-5
GRAINS		6-8
PROTEIN		3-4
DAIRY		2-3
SUGARS	FATS	moderation
VITAMINS/SUPPLEMENTS		

DAILY TOTALS:

calories

carbs   fat

protein   fiber

PHYSICAL ACTIVITY

	focus	intensity	time

COMMENTS/THOUGHTS

S M T W R F S

date   week #

FOOD LOG	calories	fat (g)	protein (g)	carbs (g)	fiber (g)
Breakfast time:					
Snack time:					
Lunch time:					
Snack time:					
Dinner time:					
Snack time:					

TODAY'S GOAL MET

MOOD

☹

2

3

4

☺

ENERGY LEVEL

🐌

2

3

4

🐇

WORKOUT RATE

great

good

okay

meh

missed

NUTRIENT TRACKER:

	# of servings	recommended
WATER		8
FRUITS		2-4
VEGETABLES		3-5
GRAINS		6-8
PROTEIN		3-4
DAIRY		2-3
SUGARS	FATS	moderation
VITAMINS/SUPPLEMENTS		

DAILY TOTALS:

calories

carbs   fat

protein   fiber

PHYSICAL ACTIVITY	focus	intensity	ti

COMMENTS/THOUGHTS

M T W R F S   date _____   week # _____

FOOD LOG

	calories	fat (g)	protein (g)	carbs (g)	fiber (g)	
breakfast time:						
snack time:						
lunch time:						
snack time:						
dinner time:						
snack time:						

TODAY'S GOAL MET

MOOD

☹
2
3
4
☺

ENERGY LEVEL

🐌
2
3
4
🐇

NUTRIENT TRACKER:

	# of servings	recommended
WATER		8
FRUITS		2-4
VEGETABLES		3-5
GRAINS		6-8
PROTEIN		3-4
DAIRY		2-3
SUGARS	FATS	moderation
VITAMINS/SUPPLEMENTS		

DAILY TOTALS:

calories

carbs   fat

protein   fiber

WORKOUT RATE

great

good

okay

meh

missed

PHYSICAL ACTIVITY

	focus	intensity	time

COMMENTS/THOUGHTS

S M T W R F S date _____ week # _____

TODAY'S GOAL MET	FOOD LOG	calories	fat (g)	protein (g)	carbs (g)	fiber (g)
	Breakfast time:					
MOOD ☹ 2 3 4 ☺	**Snack** time:					
	Lunch time:					
	Snack time:					
ENERGY LEVEL 🐌 2 3 4 🐇	**Dinner** time:					
	Snack time:					

NUTRIENT TRACKER:

	# of servings	recommended
WATER		8
FRUITS		2-4
VEGETABLES		3-5
GRAINS		6-8
PROTEIN		3-4
DAIRY		2-3
SUGARS	FATS	moderation
VITAMINS/SUPPLEMENTS		

DAILY TOTALS:

calories

carbs   fat

protein   fiber

WORKOUT RATE

great

good

okay

meh

missed

PHYSICAL ACTIVITY	focus	intensity	ti...

COMMENTS/THOUGHTS

WEEKLY WRAP-UP

date _____   week # _____

START WEIGHT

Hold on to your dreams; they will help guide you on your path to happiness.

END WEIGHT

DAYS I TRACKED MY DIET   S ▢ M ▢ T ▢ W ▢ R ▢ F ▢ S ▢

DIET NOTES

THIS WEEK'S MOOD

☹

2

3

4

☺

DAYS I EXERCISED   S ▢ M ▢ T ▢ W ▢ R ▢ F ▢ S ▢

EXERCISE NOTES

THIS WEEK'S ENERGY LEVEL

🐌

2

3

4

🐇

Did I meet this week's goals?

0%   25%   50%   75%   100%

TOTAL WORKOUT TIME

GOALS FOR NEXT WEEK

YOU CAN DO THIS!

S M T W R F S date week #

TODAY'S
GOAL MET

FOOD LOG

	calories	fat (g)	protein (g)	carbs (g)	fiber (g)
Breakfast time:					
Snack time:					
Lunch time:					
Snack time:					
Dinner time:					
Snack time:					

MOOD

☹
2
3
4
☺

ENERGY
LEVEL

🐌
2
3
4
🐇

WORKOUT
RATE

great

good

okay

meh

missed

NUTRIENT TRACKER:

	# of servings	recommended
WATER		8
FRUITS		2-4
VEGETABLES		3-5
GRAINS		6-8
PROTEIN		3-4
DAIRY		2-3
SUGARS	FATS	moderation
VITAMINS/SUPPLEMENTS		

DAILY TOTALS:

calories

carbs   fat

protein   fiber

PHYSICAL ACTIVITY

	focus	intensity	tim

COMMENTS/THOUGHTS

M T W R F S

date _____ week # _____

OOD LOG

	calories	fat (g)	protein (g)	carbs (g)	fiber (g)
reakfast ime:					
nack ime:					
unch ime:					
nack me:					
inner me:					
nack me:					

TODAY'S GOAL MET

MOOD

☹

2

3

4

☺

ENERGY LEVEL

🐌

2

3

4

🐇

WORKOUT RATE

great

good

okay

meh

missed

NUTRIENT TRACKER:

	# of servings	recommended
WATER		8
FRUITS		2-4
TABLES		3-5
GRAINS		6-8
ROTEIN		3-4
DAIRY		2-3
UGARS	FATS	moderation
AMINS/SUPPLEMENTS		

DAILY TOTALS:

calories

carbs   fat

protein   fiber

HYSICAL ACTIVITY

	focus	intensity	time

OMMENTS/THOUGHTS

S M T W R F S   date _____   week # _____

TODAY'S GOAL MET	FOOD LOG	calories	fat (g)	protein (g)	carbs (g)	fiber (g)
	Breakfast time:					
MOOD ☹ 2 3 4 ☺	**Snack** time:					
	Lunch time:					
	Snack time:					
ENERGY LEVEL 🐌 2 3 4 🐰	**Dinner** time:					
	Snack time:					

NUTRIENT TRACKER:

	# of servings	recommended
WATER		8
FRUITS		2-4
VEGETABLES		3-5
GRAINS		6-8
PROTEIN		3-4
DAIRY		2-3
SUGARS	FATS	moderation
VITAMINS/SUPPLEMENTS		

DAILY TOTALS:

calories

carbs   fat

protein   fiber

WORKOUT RATE	PHYSICAL ACTIVITY	focus	intensity	time
great				
good				
okay				
meh				
missed				

COMMENTS/THOUGHTS

S M T W R F S

date   week #

FOOD LOG

	calories	fat (g)	protein (g)	carbs (g)	fiber (g)	
Breakfast time:						
Snack time:						
Lunch time:						
Snack time:						
Dinner time:						
Snack time:						

TODAY'S GOAL ME™

MOOD

☹
2
3
4
☺

ENERGY LEVEL

🐌
2
3
4
🐇

NUTRIENT TRACKER:

	# of servings	recommended
WATER		8
FRUITS		2-4
VEGETABLES		3-5
GRAINS		6-8
PROTEIN		3-4
DAIRY		2-3
SUGARS	FATS	moderation
VITAMINS/SUPPLEMENTS		

DAILY TOTALS:

calories

carbs   fat

protein   fiber

WORKOUT RATE

great

good

okay

meh

missed

PHYSICAL ACTIVITY

	focus	intensity	time

COMMENTS/THOUGHTS

S M T W R F S   date   week

TODAY'S GOAL MET	FOOD LOG	calories	fat (g)	protein (g)	carbs (g)	fiber (g)
	Breakfast time:					
MOOD ☹ 2 3 4 ☺	**Snack** time:					
	Lunch time:					
	Snack time:					
ENERGY LEVEL 🐌 2 3 4 🐇	**Dinner** time:					
	Snack time:					

NUTRIENT TRACKER: DAILY TOTALS:

	# of servings	recommended
WATER		8
FRUITS		2-4
VEGETABLES		3-5
GRAINS		6-8
PROTEIN		3-4
DAIRY		2-3
SUGARS	FATS	moderation
VITAMINS/SUPPLEMENTS		

calories

carbs   fat

protein   fiber

WORKOUT RATE	PHYSICAL ACTIVITY	focus	intensity	time
great				
good				
okay				
meh				
missed				

COMMENTS/THOUGHTS

S M T W R F S   date   week

FOOD LOG

	calories	fat (g)	protein (g)	carbs (g)	fiber (g)	

Breakfast
time:

Snack
time:

Lunch
time:

Snack
time:

Dinner
time:

Snack
time:

TODAY'S GOAL MET

MOOD

☹
2
3
4
☺

ENERGY LEVEL

🐌
2
3
4
🐇

WORKOUT RATE

great

good

okay

meh

missed

NUTRIENT TRACKER:

of servings   recommended

	# of servings	recommended
WATER		8
FRUITS		2-4
VEGETABLES		3-5
GRAINS		6-8
PROTEIN		3-4
DAIRY		2-3
SUGARS	FATS	moderation
VITAMINS/SUPPLEMENTS		

DAILY TOTALS:

calories

carbs   fat

protein   fiber

PHYSICAL ACTIVITY

	focus	intensity	time

COMMENTS/THOUGHTS

S M T W R F S   date   week #

TODAY'S GOAL MET	FOOD LOG	calories	fat (g)	protein (g)	carbs (g)	fiber (g)
	Breakfast time:					
MOOD	**Snack** time:					
Lunch time:						
	Snack time:					
ENERGY LEVEL	**Dinner** time:					
	Snack time:					

MOOD

☹
2
3
4
☺

ENERGY LEVEL

🐌
2
3
4
🐇

NUTRIENT TRACKER:

	# of servings	recommended
WATER		8
FRUITS		2-4
VEGETABLES		3-5
GRAINS		6-8
PROTEIN		3-4
DAIRY		2-3
SUGARS	FATS	moderation
VITAMINS/SUPPLEMENTS		

DAILY TOTALS:

calories

carbs   fat

protein   fiber

WORKOUT RATE

great

good

okay

meh

missed

PHYSICAL ACTIVITY	focus	intensity	tim

COMMENTS/THOUGHTS

START WEIGHT

Be bold, and you will accomplish great things.

END WEIGHT

AYS I TRACKED MY DIET   S   M   T   W   R   F   S

IET NOTES

THIS WEEK'S MOOD

☹

2

3

4

☺

AYS I EXERCISED   S   M   T   W   R   F   S

KERCISE NOTES

THIS WEEK'S ENERGY LEVEL

🐌

2

3

4

🐇

Did I meet this week's goals?

0%   25%   50%   75%   100%

TOTAL WORKOUT TIME

OALS FOR NEXT WEEK

YOU CAN DO THIS!

S M T W R F S

date

week #

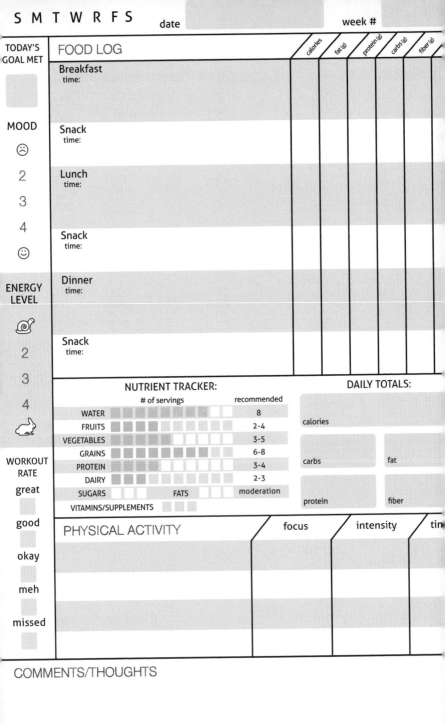

TODAY'S GOAL MET	FOOD LOG		calories	fat (g)	protein (g)	carbs (g)	fiber (g)
	Breakfast time:						
MOOD ☹	**Snack** time:						
2 3 4 ☺	**Lunch** time:						
	Snack time:						
ENERGY LEVEL 🐌 2 3 4 🐇	**Dinner** time:						
	Snack time:						

NUTRIENT TRACKER:

	# of servings	recommended
WATER		8
FRUITS		2-4
VEGETABLES		3-5
GRAINS		6-8
PROTEIN		3-4
DAIRY		2-3
SUGARS	FATS	moderation
VITAMINS/SUPPLEMENTS		

DAILY TOTALS:

calories

carbs

fat

protein

fiber

WORKOUT RATE				
great				
good				
okay				
meh				
missed				

PHYSICAL ACTIVITY	focus	intensity	tim

COMMENTS/THOUGHTS

M T W R F S   date _____   week #

FOOD LOG

	calories	fat (g)	protein (g)	carbs (g)	fiber (g)	TODAY'S GOAL MET
breakfast time:						
snack time:						**MOOD**
lunch time:						
snack time:						
dinner time:						
snack time:						

MOOD

☹
2
3
4
☺

ENERGY LEVEL

🐌
2
3
4
🐇

NUTRIENT TRACKER:

	# of servings	recommended
WATER		8
FRUITS		2-4
VEGETABLES		3-5
GRAINS		6-8
PROTEIN		3-4
DAIRY		2-3
SUGARS	FATS	moderation
VITAMINS/SUPPLEMENTS		

DAILY TOTALS:

calories

carbs   fat

protein   fiber

WORKOUT RATE

great

good

okay

meh

missed

PHYSICAL ACTIVITY

	focus	intensity	time

COMMENTS/THOUGHTS

S M T W R F S   date   week #

	FOOD LOG	calories	fat (g)	protein (g)	carbs (g)	fiber (g)
TODAY'S GOAL MET	**Breakfast** time:					
MOOD ☹ 2 3 4 ☺	**Snack** time:					
	Lunch time:					
	Snack time:					
ENERGY LEVEL 🐌 2 3 4 🐇	**Dinner** time:					
	Snack time:					

NUTRIENT TRACKER:

	# of servings	recommended
WATER		8
FRUITS		2-4
VEGETABLES		3-5
GRAINS		6-8
PROTEIN		3-4
DAIRY		2-3
SUGARS	FATS	moderation
VITAMINS/SUPPLEMENTS		

DAILY TOTALS:

calories

carbs   fat

protein   fiber

WORKOUT RATE

great

good

okay

meh

missed

PHYSICAL ACTIVITY	focus	intensity	tir

COMMENTS/THOUGHTS

S M T W R F S

date

week #

OOD LOG

	calories	fat (g)	protein (g)	carbs (g)	fiber (g)	
reakfast ime:						
nack ime:						
unch ime:						
nack me:						
inner me:						
nack ime:						

TODAY'S GOAL MET

MOOD

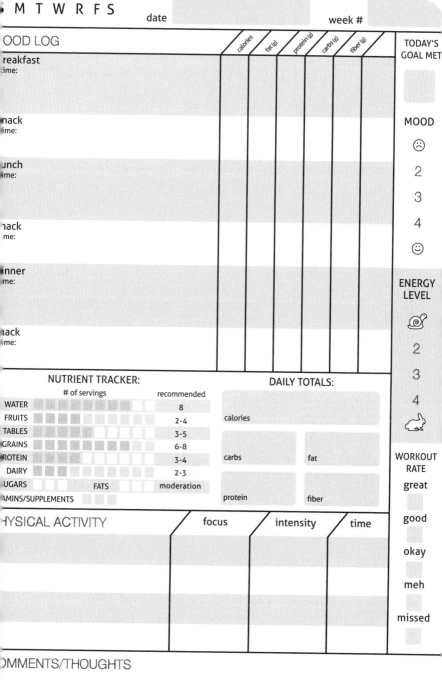

☹

2

3

4

☺

ENERGY LEVEL

🐌

2

3

4

🐰

NUTRIENT TRACKER:

	# of servings	recommended
WATER		8
FRUITS		2-4
TABLES		3-5
GRAINS		6-8
ROTEIN		3-4
DAIRY		2-3
UGARS	FATS	moderation
AMINS/SUPPLEMENTS		

DAILY TOTALS:

calories

carbs   fat

protein   fiber

WORKOUT RATE

great

good

okay

meh

missed

HYSICAL ACTIVITY

	focus	intensity	time

OMMENTS/THOUGHTS

S M T W R F S   date   week #

TODAY'S GOAL MET	FOOD LOG	calories	fat (g)	protein (g)	carbs (g)	fiber (g)
	Breakfast time:					
MOOD ☹ 2 3 4 ☺	**Snack** time:					
	Lunch time:					
	Snack time:					
ENERGY LEVEL 🐌 2 3 4 🐇	**Dinner** time:					
	Snack time:					

NUTRIENT TRACKER:

	# of servings	recommended
WATER		8
FRUITS		2-4
VEGETABLES		3-5
GRAINS		6-8
PROTEIN		3-4
DAIRY		2-3
SUGARS	FATS	moderation
VITAMINS/SUPPLEMENTS		

DAILY TOTALS:

calories

carbs   fat

protein   fiber

WORKOUT RATE	PHYSICAL ACTIVITY	focus	intensity	ti
great				
good				
okay				
meh				
missed				

COMMENTS/THOUGHTS

M T W R F S   date _____   week # _____

FOOD LOG

	calories	fat (g)	protein (g)	carbs (g)	fiber (g)	
Breakfast time:						
Snack time:						
Lunch time:						
Snack time:						
Dinner time:						
Snack time:						

TODAY'S GOAL MET

MOOD
☹
2
3
4
☺

ENERGY LEVEL
🐌
2
3
4
🐇

WORKOUT RATE
great
good
okay
meh
missed

NUTRIENT TRACKER:

	# of servings	recommended
WATER		8
FRUITS		2-4
VEGETABLES		3-5
GRAINS		6-8
PROTEIN		3-4
DAIRY		2-3
SUGARS	FATS	moderation
VITAMINS/SUPPLEMENTS		

DAILY TOTALS:

calories

carbs   fat

protein   fiber

PHYSICAL ACTIVITY

	focus	intensity	time

COMMENTS/THOUGHTS

S M T W R F S   date   week #

TODAY'S GOAL MET

FOOD LOG

	calories	fat (g)	protein (g)	carbs (g)	fiber (g)
Breakfast time:					
Snack time:					
Lunch time:					
Snack time:					
Dinner time:					
Snack time:					

MOOD

☹
2
3
4
☺

ENERGY LEVEL

🐌
2
3
4
🐇

NUTRIENT TRACKER:

	# of servings	recommended
WATER		8
FRUITS		2-4
VEGETABLES		3-5
GRAINS		6-8
PROTEIN		3-4
DAIRY		2-3
SUGARS	FATS	moderation
VITAMINS/SUPPLEMENTS		

DAILY TOTALS:

calories

carbs   fat

protein   fiber

WORKOUT RATE

great

good

okay

meh

missed

PHYSICAL ACTIVITY

	focus	intensity	tim

COMMENTS/THOUGHTS

WEEKLY WRAP-UP

date _____   week # ____

START WEIGHT

END WEIGHT

Keep your eyes on the road you travel — that is the only one you have the power to change.

DAYS I TRACKED MY DIET   S   M   T   W   R   F   S
DIET NOTES

THIS WEEK'S MOOD

☹
2
3
4
☺

DAYS I EXERCISED   S   M   T   W   R   F   S
EXERCISE NOTES

THIS WEEK'S ENERGY LEVEL

🐌
2
3
4
🐇

Did I meet this week's goals?

0%   25%   50%   75%   100%

TOTAL WORKOUT TIME

GOALS FOR NEXT WEEK

YOU CAN DO THIS!

S M T W R F S

date   week #

TODAY'S GOAL MET	FOOD LOG	calories	fat (g)	protein (g)	carbs (g)	fiber (g)
	Breakfast time:					
MOOD ☹ 2 3 4 ☺	**Snack** time:					
	Lunch time:					
	Snack time:					
ENERGY LEVEL 🐌 2 3 4 🐇	**Dinner** time:					
	Snack time:					

NUTRIENT TRACKER:

	# of servings	recommended
WATER		8
FRUITS		2-4
VEGETABLES		3-5
GRAINS		6-8
PROTEIN		3-4
DAIRY		2-3
SUGARS	FATS	moderation
VITAMINS/SUPPLEMENTS		

DAILY TOTALS:

calories

carbs   fat

protein   fiber

WORKOUT RATE

great

good

okay

meh

missed

PHYSICAL ACTIVITY	focus	intensity	tim

COMMENTS/THOUGHTS

S M T W R F S   date   week #

FOOD LOG

	calories	fat (g)	protein (g)	carbs (g)	fiber (g)	
Breakfast time:						
Snack time:						
Lunch time:						
Snack time:						
Dinner time:						
Snack time:						

TODAY'S GOAL MET

MOOD

☹

2

3

4

☺

ENERGY LEVEL

🐌

2

3

4

🐇

NUTRIENT TRACKER:

	# of servings	recommended
WATER		8
FRUITS		2-4
VEGETABLES		3-5
GRAINS		6-8
PROTEIN		3-4
DAIRY		2-3
SUGARS	FATS	moderation
VITAMINS/SUPPLEMENTS		

DAILY TOTALS:

calories

carbs   fat

protein   fiber

WORKOUT RATE

great

good

okay

meh

missed

PHYSICAL ACTIVITY

	focus	intensity	time

COMMENTS/THOUGHTS

S M T W R F S

date _____   week # _____

	FOOD LOG	calories	fat (g)	protein (g)	carbs (g)	fiber (g)	

TODAY'S GOAL MET

Breakfast
time:

MOOD

☹

2

3

4

☺

Snack
time:

Lunch
time:

Snack
time:

ENERGY LEVEL

🐌

2

3

4

🐰

Dinner
time:

Snack
time:

NUTRIENT TRACKER:

	# of servings	recommended
WATER		8
FRUITS		2-4
VEGETABLES		3-5
GRAINS		6-8
PROTEIN		3-4
DAIRY		2-3
SUGARS	FATS	moderation
VITAMINS/SUPPLEMENTS		

DAILY TOTALS:

calories

carbs   fat

protein   fiber

WORKOUT RATE

great

good

okay

meh

missed

PHYSICAL ACTIVITY	focus	intensity	tin

COMMENTS/THOUGHTS

S M T W R F S   date   week #

FOOD LOG

	calories	fat (g)	protein (g)	carbs (g)	fiber (g)	
breakfast time:						
snack time:						
lunch time:						
snack time:						
dinner time:						
snack time:						

TODAY'S GOAL MET

MOOD

☹
2
3
4
☺

ENERGY LEVEL

🐌
2
3
4
🐇

NUTRIENT TRACKER:

	# of servings	recommended
WATER		8
FRUITS		2-4
VEGETABLES		3-5
GRAINS		6-8
PROTEIN		3-4
DAIRY		2-3
SUGARS	FATS	moderation
VITAMINS/SUPPLEMENTS		

DAILY TOTALS:

calories

carbs   fat

protein   fiber

WORKOUT RATE

great

good

okay

meh

missed

PHYSICAL ACTIVITY

	focus	intensity	time

COMMENTS/THOUGHTS

S M T W R F S   date   week #

TODAY'S GOAL MET	FOOD LOG	calories	fat (g)	protein (g)	carbs (g)	fiber (g)
	Breakfast time:					
MOOD ☹ 2 3 4 ☺	**Snack** time:					
	Lunch time:					
	Snack time:					
ENERGY LEVEL 🐌 2 3 4 🐇	**Dinner** time:					
	Snack time:					

NUTRIENT TRACKER:

	# of servings	recommended
WATER		8
FRUITS		2-4
VEGETABLES		3-5
GRAINS		6-8
PROTEIN		3-4
DAIRY		2-3
SUGARS	FATS	moderation
VITAMINS/SUPPLEMENTS		

DAILY TOTALS:

calories

carbs   fat

protein   fiber

WORKOUT RATE

great

good

okay

meh

missed

PHYSICAL ACTIVITY	focus	intensity	tin

COMMENTS/THOUGHTS

S M T W R F S date [   ] week #

OOD LOG

	calories	fat (g)	protein (g)	carbs (g)	fiber (g)	

reakfast
ime:

nack
ime:

unch
ime:

nack
me:

inner
me:

nack
me:

NUTRIENT TRACKER:

	# of servings	recommended
WATER		8
FRUITS		2-4
TABLES		3-5
GRAINS		6-8
ROTEIN		3-4
DAIRY		2-3
UGARS	FATS	moderation
AMINS/SUPPLEMENTS		

DAILY TOTALS:

calories

carbs | fat

protein | fiber

TODAY'S GOAL MET

MOOD

☹

2

3

4

☺

ENERGY LEVEL

🐌

2

3

4

🐇

WORKOUT RATE

great

good

okay

meh

missed

HYSICAL ACTIVITY

	focus	intensity	time

OMMENTS/THOUGHTS

S M T W R F S   date _____   week # _____

TODAY'S GOAL MET	FOOD LOG	calories	fat (g)	protein (g)	carbs (g)	fiber (g)
	Breakfast time:					
MOOD ☹ 2 3 4 ☺	**Snack** time:					
	Lunch time:					
	Snack time:					
ENERGY LEVEL 🐌 2 3 4 🐰	**Dinner** time:					
	Snack time:					

NUTRIENT TRACKER:

	# of servings	recommended
WATER		8
FRUITS		2-4
VEGETABLES		3-5
GRAINS		6-8
PROTEIN		3-4
DAIRY		2-3
SUGARS	FATS	moderation
VITAMINS/SUPPLEMENTS		

DAILY TOTALS:

calories

carbs   fat

protein   fiber

WORKOUT RATE

great

good

okay

meh

missed

PHYSICAL ACTIVITY	focus	intensity	tim

COMMENTS/THOUGHTS

WEEKLY WRAP-UP

date _____   week # _____

	START WEIGHT

Happiness is a day-to-day choice,
not a by-product of circumstances.

END WEIGHT

DAYS I TRACKED MY DIET   S   M   T   W   R   F   S

DIET NOTES

THIS WEEK'S MOOD

☹

2

3

4

☺

DAYS I EXERCISED   S   M   T   W   R   F   S

EXERCISE NOTES

THIS WEEK'S ENERGY LEVEL

🐌

2

3

4

🐇

Did I meet this week's goals?

0%   25%   50%   75%   100%

TOTAL WORKOUT TIME

GOALS FOR NEXT WEEK

YOU CAN DO THIS!

S M T W R F S   date ____   week # ____

TODAY'S GOAL MET	FOOD LOG	calories	fat (g)	protein (g)	carbs (g)	fiber (g)
	Breakfast time:					
MOOD ☹ 2 3 4 ☺	**Snack** time:					
	Lunch time:					
	Snack time:					
ENERGY LEVEL 🐌 2 3 4 🐇	**Dinner** time:					
	Snack time:					

NUTRIENT TRACKER:

	# of servings	recommended
WATER		8
FRUITS		2-4
VEGETABLES		3-5
GRAINS		6-8
PROTEIN		3-4
DAIRY		2-3
SUGARS	FATS	moderation
VITAMINS/SUPPLEMENTS		

DAILY TOTALS:

calories

carbs   fat

protein   fiber

WORKOUT RATE

great

good

okay

meh

missed

PHYSICAL ACTIVITY	focus	intensity	tin

COMMENTS/THOUGHTS

S M T W R F S   date ____   week # ____

FOOD LOG

	calories	fat (g)	protein (g)	carbs (g)	fiber (g)	

breakfast
time:

snack
time:

lunch
time:

snack
time:

dinner
time:

snack
time:

NUTRIENT TRACKER:

	# of servings	recommended
WATER		8
FRUITS		2-4
VEGETABLES		3-5
GRAINS		6-8
PROTEIN		3-4
DAIRY		2-3
SUGARS	FATS	moderation
VITAMINS/SUPPLEMENTS		

DAILY TOTALS:

calories

carbs   fat

protein   fiber

PHYSICAL ACTIVITY

	focus	intensity	time

TODAY'S GOAL MET

MOOD

☹
2
3
4
☺

ENERGY LEVEL

🐌
2
3
4
🐇

WORKOUT RATE

great

good

okay

meh

missed

COMMENTS/THOUGHTS

S M T W R F S   date   week

FOOD LOG

TODAY'S GOAL MET	FOOD LOG	calories	fat (g)	protein (g)	carbs (g)	fiber (g)
	Breakfast time:					
MOOD ☹ 2 3 4 ☺	**Snack** time:					
	Lunch time:					
	Snack time:					
ENERGY LEVEL 🐌 2 3 4 🐇	**Dinner** time:					
	Snack time:					

NUTRIENT TRACKER:

	# of servings	recommended
WATER		8
FRUITS		2-4
VEGETABLES		3-5
GRAINS		6-8
PROTEIN		3-4
DAIRY		2-3
SUGARS	FATS	moderation
VITAMINS/SUPPLEMENTS		

DAILY TOTALS:

calories

carbs   fat

protein   fiber

WORKOUT RATE
great
good
okay
meh
missed

PHYSICAL ACTIVITY	focus	intensity	tim

COMMENTS/THOUGHTS

OOD LOG

	calories	fat (g)	protein (g)	carbs (g)	fiber (g)	
reakfast ime:						
nack ime:						
unch ime:						
nack ime:						
inner ime:						
ack ime:						

TODAY'S GOAL MET

MOOD
🙁
2
3
4
☺

ENERGY LEVEL
🐌
2
3
4
🐇

NUTRIENT TRACKER:

	# of servings	recommended
WATER		8
FRUITS		2-4
ETABLES		3-5
GRAINS		6-8
PROTEIN		3-4
DAIRY		2-3
SUGARS	FATS	moderation
AMINS/SUPPLEMENTS		

DAILY TOTALS:

calories

carbs   fat

protein   fiber

WORKOUT RATE

great

good

okay

meh

missed

HYSICAL ACTIVITY

	focus	intensity	time

OMMENTS/THOUGHTS

S M T W R F S   date   week #

TODAY'S GOAL MET	FOOD LOG	calories	fat (g)	protein (g)	carbs (g)	fiber (g)
	Breakfast time:					
MOOD	**Snack** time:					
☹ 2 3 4 ☺	**Lunch** time:					
	Snack time:					
ENERGY LEVEL	**Dinner** time:					
🐌 2 3 4 🐰	**Snack** time:					

NUTRIENT TRACKER:

	# of servings	recommended
WATER		8
FRUITS		2-4
VEGETABLES		3-5
GRAINS		6-8
PROTEIN		3-4
DAIRY		2-3
SUGARS	FATS	moderation
VITAMINS/SUPPLEMENTS		

DAILY TOTALS:

calories

carbs   fat

protein   fiber

WORKOUT RATE

great

good

okay

meh

missed

PHYSICAL ACTIVITY	focus	intensity	tim

COMMENTS/THOUGHTS

S M T W R F S   date   week #

FOOD LOG

	calories	fat (g)	protein (g)	carbs (g)	fiber (g)		TODAY'S GOAL MET
breakfast time:							
snack time:							MOOD
lunch time:							☹ 2 3 4 ☺
snack time:							
dinner time:							ENERGY LEVEL
snack time:							

NUTRIENT TRACKER:

	# of servings	recommended
WATER		8
FRUITS		2-4
TABLES		3-5
GRAINS		6-8
PROTEIN		3-4
DAIRY		2-3
UGARS	FATS	moderation
AMINS/SUPPLEMENTS		

DAILY TOTALS:

calories

carbs   fat

protein   fiber

ENERGY LEVEL

🐌 2 3 4 🐇

WORKOUT RATE

great

good

okay

meh

missed

PHYSICAL ACTIVITY

	focus	intensity	time

COMMENTS/THOUGHTS

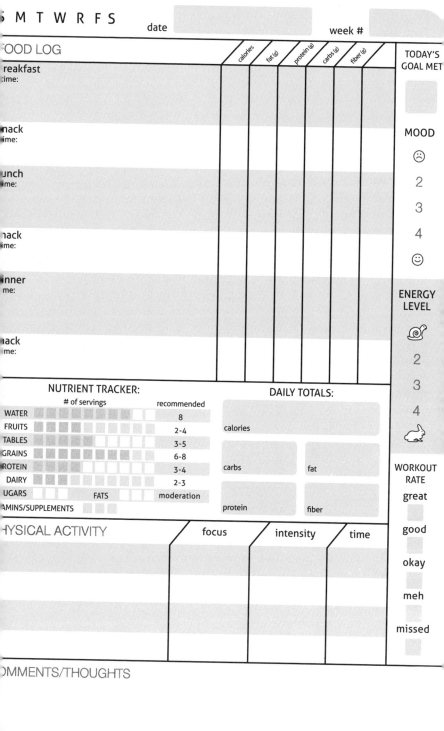

S M T W R F S   date   week

	FOOD LOG	calories	fat (g)	protein (g)	carbs (g)	fiber (g)

TODAY'S GOAL MET

Breakfast
time:

MOOD

☹

2

3

4

☺

Snack
time:

Lunch
time:

Snack
time:

ENERGY LEVEL

🐌

2

3

4

🐇

Dinner
time:

Snack
time:

NUTRIENT TRACKER:

DAILY TOTALS:

	# of servings	recommended
WATER		8
FRUITS		2-4
VEGETABLES		3-5
GRAINS		6-8
PROTEIN		3-4
DAIRY		2-3
SUGARS	FATS	moderation
VITAMINS/SUPPLEMENTS		

calories

carbs   fat

protein   fiber

WORKOUT RATE

great

good

okay

meh

missed

PHYSICAL ACTIVITY	focus	intensity	tim

COMMENTS/THOUGHTS

WEEKLY WRAP-UP

date _____ week # _____

> Time well spent is the best investment we can ever make, and it doesn't cost a thing.

START WEIGHT

END WEIGHT

DAYS I TRACKED MY DIET S M T W R F S

DIET NOTES

THIS WEEK'S MOOD

☹
2
3
4
☺

DAYS I EXERCISED S M T W R F S

EXERCISE NOTES

THIS WEEK'S ENERGY LEVEL

🐌
2
3
4
🐇

Did I meet this week's goals?

0%   25%   50%   75%   100%

TOTAL WORKOUT TIME

GOALS FOR NEXT WEEK

YOU CAN DO THIS!

S M T W R F S   date   week

<table>
<tr><td colspan="2"></td><td>calories</td><td>fat (g)</td><td>protein (g)</td><td>carbs (g)</td><td>fiber (g)</td></tr>
</table>

TODAY'S GOAL MET

FOOD LOG

	calories	fat (g)	protein (g)	carbs (g)	fiber (g)
Breakfast time:					
Snack time:					
Lunch time:					
Snack time:					
Dinner time:					
Snack time:					

MOOD

☹

2

3

4

☺

ENERGY LEVEL

🐌

2

3

4

🐰

WORKOUT RATE

great

good

okay

meh

missed

NUTRIENT TRACKER:

	# of servings	recommended
WATER		8
FRUITS		2-4
VEGETABLES		3-5
GRAINS		6-8
PROTEIN		3-4
DAIRY		2-3
SUGARS	FATS	moderation
VITAMINS/SUPPLEMENTS		

DAILY TOTALS:

calories

carbs

fat

protein

fiber

PHYSICAL ACTIVITY

	focus	intensity	time

COMMENTS/THOUGHTS

S M T W R F S   date _____   week # ____

FOOD LOG

	calories	fat (g)	protein (g)	carbs (g)	fiber (g)
breakfast time:					
snack time:					
lunch time:					
snack time:					
dinner time:					
snack time:					

TODAY'S GOAL MET

MOOD

☹

2

3

4

☺

ENERGY LEVEL

🐌

2

3

4

🐇

WORKOUT RATE

great

good

okay

meh

missed

NUTRIENT TRACKER:

	# of servings	recommended
WATER		8
FRUITS		2-4
VEGETABLES		3-5
GRAINS		6-8
PROTEIN		3-4
DAIRY		2-3
SUGARS	FATS	moderation
VITAMINS/SUPPLEMENTS		

DAILY TOTALS:

calories

carbs   fat

protein   fiber

PHYSICAL ACTIVITY

	focus	intensity	time

COMMENTS/THOUGHTS

S M T W R F S   date _____   week # _____

	FOOD LOG	calories	fat (g)	protein (g)	carbs (g)	fiber (g)
TODAY'S GOAL MET	**Breakfast** time:					
MOOD ☹ 2 3 4 ☺	**Snack** time:					
	Lunch time:					
	Snack time:					
ENERGY LEVEL 🐌 2 3 4 🐇	**Dinner** time:					
	Snack time:					

NUTRIENT TRACKER:

	# of servings	recommended
WATER		8
FRUITS		2-4
VEGETABLES		3-5
GRAINS		6-8
PROTEIN		3-4
DAIRY		2-3
SUGARS	FATS	moderation
VITAMINS/SUPPLEMENTS		

DAILY TOTALS:

calories

carbs   fat

protein   fiber

WORKOUT RATE

great

good

okay

meh

missed

PHYSICAL ACTIVITY	focus	intensity	tir

COMMENTS/THOUGHTS

S M T W R F S   date   week #

FOOD LOG	calories	fat (g)	protein (g)	carbs (g)	fiber (g)		TODAY'S GOAL MET
Breakfast time:							
Snack time:							**MOOD** ☹
Lunch time:							2
							3
							4
Snack time:							☺
Dinner time:							**ENERGY LEVEL** 🐌
Snack time:							2

NUTRIENT TRACKER:

	# of servings	recommended
WATER		8
FRUITS		2-4
VEGETABLES		3-5
GRAINS		6-8
PROTEIN		3-4
DAIRY		2-3
SUGARS	FATS	moderation
VITAMINS/SUPPLEMENTS		

DAILY TOTALS:

calories

carbs   fat

protein   fiber

3
4
🐇

PHYSICAL ACTIVITY	focus	intensity	time	WORKOUT RATE
				great
				good
				okay
				meh
				missed

COMMENTS/THOUGHTS

S M T W R F S   date _____   week # _____

	FOOD LOG		calories	fat (g)	protein (g)	carbs (g)	fiber (g)

TODAY'S GOAL MET

Breakfast
time:

MOOD
☹
2
3
4
☺

Snack
time:

Lunch
time:

Snack
time:

ENERGY LEVEL
🐌
2
3
4
🐰

Dinner
time:

Snack
time:

NUTRIENT TRACKER:

	# of servings	recommended
WATER		8
FRUITS		2-4
VEGETABLES		3-5
GRAINS		6-8
PROTEIN		3-4
DAIRY		2-3
SUGARS	FATS	moderation
VITAMINS/SUPPLEMENTS		

DAILY TOTALS:

calories

carbs   fat

protein   fiber

WORKOUT RATE
great
good
okay
meh
missed

PHYSICAL ACTIVITY	focus	intensity	tim...

COMMENTS/THOUGHTS

S M T W R F S

date

week #

FOOD LOG

	calories	fat (g)	protein (g)	carbs (g)	fiber (g)

Breakfast
time:

Snack
time:

Lunch
time:

Snack
time:

Dinner
time:

Snack
time:

TODAY'S GOAL MET

MOOD

☹
2
3
4
☺

ENERGY LEVEL

🐌
2
3
4
🐇

NUTRIENT TRACKER:

	# of servings	recommended
WATER		8
FRUITS		2-4
VEGETABLES		3-5
GRAINS		6-8
PROTEIN		3-4
DAIRY		2-3
SUGARS	FATS	moderation
VITAMINS/SUPPLEMENTS		

DAILY TOTALS:

calories

carbs | fat

protein | fiber

WORKOUT RATE

great

good

okay

meh

missed

PHYSICAL ACTIVITY

	focus	intensity	time

COMMENTS/THOUGHTS

S M T W R F S   date   week #

	FOOD LOG	calories	fat (g)	protein (g)	carbs (g)	fiber (g)
TODAY'S GOAL MET	**Breakfast** time:					
MOOD ☹ 2 3 4 ☺	**Snack** time:					
	Lunch time:					
	Snack time:					
ENERGY LEVEL 🐌 2 3 4 🐇	**Dinner** time:					
	Snack time:					

NUTRIENT TRACKER:

	# of servings	recommended
WATER		8
FRUITS		2-4
VEGETABLES		3-5
GRAINS		6-8
PROTEIN		3-4
DAIRY		2-3
SUGARS	FATS	moderation
VITAMINS/SUPPLEMENTS		

DAILY TOTALS:

calories

carbs   fat

protein   fiber

WORKOUT RATE

great

good

okay

meh

missed

PHYSICAL ACTIVITY	focus	intensity	tin

COMMENTS/THOUGHTS

WEEKLY WRAP-UP

date

week #

START WEIGHT

Nothing great was ever accomplished
by sitting in the stands.

END WEIGHT

DAYS I TRACKED MY DIET   S   M   T   W   R   F   S

DIET NOTES

THIS WEEK'S MOOD

☹

2

3

4

☺

DAYS I EXERCISED   S   M   T   W   R   F   S

EXERCISE NOTES

THIS WEEK'S ENERGY LEVEL

🐌

2

3

4

🐰

Did I meet this week's goals?

TOTAL WORKOUT TIME

0%   25%   50%   75%   100%

GOALS FOR NEXT WEEK

YOU CAN DO THIS!

NUTRITION CHART

This nutrient counter was adapted from: U.S. Department of Agriculture, Agricultural Research Service. 2011. USDA Nutrient Database for Standard Reference, Release 16. Nutrient Data Laboratory Home Page, http://www.nal.usda.gov/fnic/foodcomp.

FOOD	CALORIES	FAT (g)	PROTEIN (g)	CARBS (g)	FIBER (g)
Almonds, 1 cup, whole	827	72	30	28	17
Anchovy, European, canned in oil, drained, 1 anchovy	8	Tr	1	0	0
Apple juice, unsweetened, 1 cup	117	Tr	Tr	29	Tr
Apple pie, 1 slice	277	13	2	40	2
Apples, raw, with skin, 1 medium	72	Tr	Tr	19	3
Applesauce, sweetened, 1 cup	194	Tr	Tr	51	3
Apricot, raw	17	Tr	Tr	4	1
Apricots, dried, stewed, without added sugar, halves, 1 cup	213	Tr	3	55	7
Apricots, juice pack, with skin, halves, 1 cup	117	Tr	2	30	4
Artichoke hearts, boiled, ½ cup	42	Tr	3	9	5
Asparagus, boiled, 4 spears	13	Tr	1	2	1
Avocados, raw, 1 cup, puréed	368	34	5	20	15
Bacon, cured, pan-fried, 1 slice	42	3	3	Tr	0
Bacon, meatless, 1 strip	16	1	1	Tr	Tr
Bagel, plain, 1 medium	270	2	11	53	2
Bamboo shoots, boiled, 1 cup	14	Tr	2	2	1
Banana chips, 1 oz.	147	10	1	17	2
Banana, raw, 1 medium	105	Tr	1	27	3
Bass, striped, cooked, 3 oz.	105	3	19	0	0
Beans, baked, canned, plain or vegetarian, 1 cup	236	1	12	52	13
Beans, black, boiled, 1 cup	227	1	15	41	15
Beans, kidney, boiled, 1 cup	225	1	15	40	11
Beans, lima, canned, ½ cup	88	Tr	5	17	4
Beans, navy, boiled, 1 cup	258	1	16	48	12
Beans, snap, green, boiled, 1 cup	44	Tr	2	10	4
Beef jerky, 1 piece, large	82	5	7	2	Tr
Beef, cured, sausage, cooked, smoked, 1 sausage	134	12	6	1	0
Beef, ground, 95% lean, ¼ lb. raw	140	5	22	0	0
Beets, boiled, slices, ½ cup	37	Tr	1	8	2

* Tr= trace amounts

FOOD	CALORIES	FAT (g)	PROTEIN (g)	CARBS (g)	FIBER (g)
Blackberries, raw, 1 cup	62	1	2	14	8
Blueberries, raw, 1 cup	83	Tr	1	21	3
Bologna, beef, 1 oz. slice	87	8	3	1	0
Bologna, turkey, 1 slice	59	4	3	1	Tr
Bran flakes, ¾ cup	96	1	3	24	5
Bratwurst, pork, cooked, 1 link	281	25	12	2	0
Brazilnuts, dried, unblanched, 1 cup shelled	918	93	20	17	11
Bread, mixed-grain, 1 slice	65	1	3	12	2
Bread, pita, whole-wheat, 1 small	74	1	3	15	2
Bread, white, 1 slice	80	1	2	15	1
Bread, whole-wheat, 1 slice	80	1	3	15	3
Brisket, whole, braised, 3 oz.	327	27	20	0	0
Broccoli, raw, 1 cup chopped	30	Tr	2	6	2
Brownies, 2" square	227	9	3	36	1
Brussels sprouts, boiled, 1 sprout	8	Tr	1	1	1
Cabbage, raw, shredded, 1 cup	17	Tr	1	4	2
Canadian-style bacon, cured, grilled, 2 slices	87	4	11	1	0
Cantaloupe, raw, ⅛ melon	23	Tr	1	6	1
Caramels, 1 piece	39	1	Tr	8	Tr
Carbonated beverage, diet or sugar-free, 12 fl. oz.	0	0	Tr	0	0
Carrots, baby, raw, 1 small	4	Tr	Tr	1	Tr
Carrots, raw, 1 medium	25	Tr	1	6	2
Cashew nuts, dry-roasted, with salt added, 1 cup	786	63	21	45	4
Catfish, cooked, 3 oz.	89	2	16	0	0
Catsup, 1 tbsp	14	Tr	Tr	4	Tr
Cauliflower, boiled, ½ cup	14	Tr	1	3	2
Cauliflower, raw, 1 floweret	3	Tr	Tr	1	Tr
Celery, raw, 1 medium stalk	6	Tr	Tr	1	1
Cheese, blue, 1 oz.	100	8	6	1	0
Cheese, brie, 1 oz.	95	8	6	Tr	0
Cheese, cheddar or colby, 1 oz.	114	9	7	Tr	0
Cheese, cottage, low-fat, 1% milkfat, 1 cup	163	2	28	6	0
Cheese, cream, 1 tbsp	51	5	1	Tr	0

FOOD	CALORIES	FAT (g)	PROTEIN (g)	CARBS (g)	FIBER (g)
Cheese, feta, crumbled, 1 cup	396	32	21	6	0
Cheese, low-fat, cheddar or colby, 1 oz.	49	2	7	1	0
Cheese, mozzarella, part skim, 1 oz.	72	5	7	1	0
Cheese, parmesan, grated, 1 tbsp	22	1	2	Tr	0
Cheese, provolone, 1 oz.	98	7	7	1	0
Cheese, ricotta, part skim, ½ cup	171	10	14	6	0
Cheese, swiss, 1oz.	108	8	8	2	0
Cheeseburger, single patty, with condiments, 1 sandwich	295	14	16	27	na
Cheesecake	257	18	4	20	Tr
Cherries, sweet, raw, 1 cherry	4	Tr	Tr	1	Tr
Chicken fillet sandwich, plain, 1 sandwich	515	29	24	39	na
Chicken, breast, meat and skin, roasted, ½ breast	193	8	29	0	0
Chicken, canned, no broth, 5 oz. can	230	10	32	1	0
Chicken, drumstick, meat and skin, roasted, 1 drumstick	112	6	14	0	0
Chicken, roasted, light meat only, 1 cup chopped	214	6	38	0	0
Chickpeas (garbanzo beans), boiled, 1 cup	269	4	15	45	12
Chili con carne, 8 fl. oz.	256	8	25	22	na
Chili with beans, canned, 1 cup	287	14	15	30	11
Chocolate Cake, without frosting	340	14	5	51	2
Chocolate chip cookie	190	9	2	26	1
Citrus fruit juice drink, frozen concentrate, 8 fl. oz.	124	Tr	Tr	30	Tr
Clam, raw, 1 medium	11	Tr	2	Tr	0
Club soda, 12 fl. oz.	0	0	0	0	0
Cocoa mix, powder, 3 heaping tsp	111	1	2	24	1
Cod, Atlantic, cooked, 3 oz.	70	1	15	0	0
Coffee, brewed from grounds, 8 fl. oz.	2	0	Tr	0	0
Cola, carbonated, 12 fl. oz.	155	0	Tr	40	0
Coleslaw, ½ cup	41	2	1	7	1
Collards, boiled, chopped, 1 cup	49	1	4	9	5
Corn chips, plain, 1 bag (7 oz.)	1067	66	13	113	10
Corn grits, cooked with water, 1 cup	143	Tr	3	31	1
Corn tortilla	62	1	2	13	2
Corn, sweet, boiled, 1 ear	83	1	3	19	2

FOOD	CALORIES	FAT (g)	PROTEIN (g)	CARBS (g)	FIBER (g)
Corn, sweet, canned, whole kernel, 1 cup	133	2	4	30	3
Corned beef, brisket, cured, cooked, 3 oz.	213	16	15	Tr	0
Couscous, cooked, 1 cup	176	Tr	6	36	2
Crab cake, 1 cake	160	10	11	5	Tr
Crackers, matzo, plain	111	Tr	3	23	1
Crackers, saltines, 1 cracker	13	Tr	Tr	2	Tr
Crackers, wheat, 1 thin square	9	Tr	Tr	1	Tr
Crackers, whole-wheat, 1 cracker	18	1	Tr	3	Tr
Cranberry juice cocktail, 8 fl. oz.	144	Tr	0	36	Tr
Cranberry sauce, canned, sweetened, 1 slice	86	Tr	Tr	22	1
Cream, half-and-half, 1 tbsp	20	2	Tr	1	0
Cream, sour, 1 tbsp	26	3	Tr	1	0
Croissants, butter	231	12	5	26	1
Croutons, ½ cup	93	4	2	13	1
Cucumber, ½ cup slices	8	Tr	Tr	2	Tr
Danish pastry, fruit,	263	13	4	34	1
Date, medjool	66	Tr	Tr	18	2
Doughnut, cake, plain, frosted	204	13	2	21	1
Duck, roasted,½ duck	1287	108	73	0	0
Egg substitute, liquid, ¼ cup	29	0	6	1	0
Egg, whole, fried or scrambled, 1 large	92	7	6	Tr	0
Egg, whole, hard-boiled	78	5	6	0	0
Eggplant, boiled, 1 cup cubes	35	Tr	1	9	2
Enchilada, cheese and beef, 1 enchilada	323	18	12	30	na
English muffin, enriched	134	1	4	26	2
Fig, raw	37	Tr	Tr	10	1
Fish fillet, battered or breaded, fried, 1 fillet	211	11	13	15	Tr
Fish sandwich, with tartar sauce, 1 sandwich	431	23	17	41	na
Fish sticks, frozen, preheated, 1 stick	76	3	4	7	Tr
Flatfish (flounder and sole), cooked, 1 fillet	149	2	31	0	0
Flour tortillas	150	3	4	26	2
French fries, in vegetable oil, 1 small order	291	16	4	34	3
French toast, made with low-fat (2%) milk	149	7	5	16	na

FOOD	CALORIES	FAT (g)	PROTEIN (g)	CARBS (g)	FIBER (g)
Frozen juice novelties, fruit and juice bars, 1 bar	63	Tr	1	16	1
Frozen yogurt, soft-serve, ½ cup (4 fl. oz.)	116	4	3	18	2
Fruit cocktail, juice pack, 1 cup	109	Tr	1	28	2
Gelatin dessert, dry mix, prepared with water, ½ cup	84	0	2	19	0
Ginger ale, 12 fl. oz.	124	0	0	32	0
Graham crackers, 1 square	30	1	Tr	5	Tr
Granola bar, hard, peanut, 1 oz.	136	6	3	18	1
Granola bar, soft, uncoated, nut and raisin, 1 bar (1 oz.)	127	6	2	18	2
Grape juice, 8 fl. oz.	150	0	Tr	37	na
Grape juice, sweetened, 1 cup	128	Tr	Tr	32	Tr
Grapefruit juice, white, canned, sweetened, 1 cup	115	Tr	1	28	Tr
Grapefruit, raw, ½ medium	41	Tr	1	10	1
Grapes, red or green, raw, seedless, 1 grape	3	Tr	Tr	1	Tr
Gravy, beef or brown, 1 serving	25	1	1	4	Tr
Ground pork, cooked, 3 oz.	252	18	22	0	0
Gumdrops, 10 gummy bears	87	0	0	22	Tr
Halibut, cooked, 3 oz.	119	2	23	0	0
Ham, cured, boneless, extra-lean, roasted, 3 oz.	123	5	18	1	0
Hamburger, single patty, with condiments, 1 sandwich	272	10	12	34	2
Hazelnuts, 10 nuts	88	9	2	2	1
Honey, 1 tbsp	64	0	Tr	17	Tr
Honeydew, melon, 1 slice	45	Tr	1	11	1
Hotdog, plain, on bun	242	15	10	18	na
Hummus, 1 tbsp	27	1	1	3	1
Ice cream, low-fat, chocolate, vanilla, or strawberry, ½ cup	143	5	3	19	1
Ice milk, vanilla, soft-serve, with cone, 1 cone	164	6	4	24	Tr
Jams, jellies, and preserves, 1 tbsp	56	Tr	Tr	14	Tr
Kaiser, 1 roll	167	2	6	30	1
Kale, cooked, chopped, 1 cup	36	1	2	7	3
Kiwi fruit, skinless, 1 medium	46	Tr	1	11	2
Lamb, ground, broiled, 3 oz.	241	17	21	0	0
Lamb, leg (shank and sirloin), roasted, 3 oz.	219	14	22	0	0
Lemonade, low-calorie, powder, 8 fl. oz.	5	0	Tr	1	0

FOOD	CALORIES	FAT (g)	PROTEIN (g)	CARBS (g)	FIBER (g)
Lentils, boiled, 1 cup	230	1	18	40	16
Lettuce, butterhead or iceberg, 1 leaf	1	Tr	Tr	Tr	Tr
Lettuce, cos or romaine, 1 leaf	2	Tr	Tr	Tr	Tr
Macadamia nuts, dry-roasted, 1 oz.	203	22	2	4	2
Macaroni, cooked, enriched, 1 cup	220	1	7	45	2
Macaroni, whole-wheat, cooked, 1 cup	174	1	7	37	4
Mangos, raw, 1 fruit	135	1	1	35	4
Margarine, stick or tub, 80% fat, 1 tbsp	100	11	Tr	Tr	0
Marshmallows, 1 regular	23	Tr	Tr	6	Tr
Milk chocolate, 1 bar	235	13	3	26	1
Milk, 2%, 1 cup	122	5	8	11	0
Milk, fat-free or skim, 1 cup	83	Tr	8	12	0
Muffins, blueberry, 1 medium	313	7	6	54	3
Mushrooms, raw, 1 medium	4	Tr	1	1	Tr
Nectarine, raw	60	Tr	1	14	2
Noodles, egg, cooked, 1 cup	213	2	8	40	2
Oats, 1 cup	607	11	26	103	17
Oats, instant, prepared with water, cooked, 1 cup	129	2	5	22	4
Oil (olive, peanut, sesame, soybean), 1 tbsp	120	14	0	0	0
Oil, vegetable (canola, corn, safflower, sunflower), 1 tbsp	120	15	0	0	0
Okra, boiled, ½ cup slices	18	Tr	1	4	2
Olives, ripe, canned, 1 large	5	Tr	Tr	Tr	Tr
Onion rings, breaded and fried, (8–9 onion rings)	276	16	4	31	na
Onion rings, breaded, pan-fried, 10 rings	244	16	3	23	1
Orange juice, canned, unsweetened, 1 cup	105	Tr	1	25	Tr
Orange roughy, 3 oz., cooked	59	1	12	0	0
Oranges, raw, 1 medium	62	Tr	1	15	3
Oyster, Eastern, breaded/fried, 6 medium	173	11	8	10	0
Pancake	74	1	2	14	Tr
Pastrami, cured, 1 slice (1 oz.)	98	8	5	1	0
Peach, raw	58	Tr	1	14	2
Peaches, canned, juice pack, halves or slices, 1 cup	109	Tr	2	29	3
Peanut bar, 1 bar	209	13	6	19	2

FOOD	CALORIES	FAT (g)	PROTEIN (g)	CARBS (g)	FIBER (g)
Peanut butter, chunky or smooth, 2 tbsp	190	16	8	7	2
Peanuts, dry-roasted, without salt, 1 cup	854	73	35	31	12
Pear, raw	96	Tr	1	26	5
Pears, canned, juice pack, with liquid	38	Tr	Tr	10	1
Peas and carrots, boiled, ½ cup	38	Tr	2	8	2
Peas, green, boiled, 1 cup	134	Tr	9	25	9
Peas, split, boiled, 1 cup	231	1	16	41	16
Pecans, 1 oz. (20 halves)	196	20	3	4	3
Pepperoni, pork/beef, 15 slices	135	12	6	1	Tr
Peppers, jalapeno, 1 pepper	4	Tr	Tr	1	Tr
Peppers, sweet, green, raw, 1 medium	24	Tr	1	6	2
Perch or Pike, cooked, 3 oz.	99	1	21	0	0
Pickle relish, 1 tbsp	14	Tr	Tr	4	Tr
Pickle, dill, 1 medium	12	Tr	Tr	3	1
Pickle, sweet, 1 midget gherkin	7	Tr	Tr	2	Tr
Pine nuts, dried, 10 nuts	11	1	Tr	Tr	Tr
Pineapple and grapefruit juice, canned, 8 fl. oz.	118	Tr	1	29	Tr
Pineapple and orange juice, canned, 8 fl. oz.	125	0	3	30	Tr
Pineapple juice, canned, unsweetened, 1 cup	140	Tr	1	34	1
Pineapple, canned, 1 cup, crushed, sliced, or chunks	149	Tr	1	39	2
Pineapple, raw, 1 slice	40	Tr	Tr	11	1
Pistachio nuts, dry-roasted, without salt added, 1 cup	702	57	26	34	13
Pizza with cheese, 1 slice	140	3	8	21	na
Pizza with cheese, meat, and vegetables, 1 slice	184	5	13	21	na
Plantain, raw	218	1	2	57	4
Plum, raw	30	Tr	Tr	8	1
Popcorn, air-popped, 1 cup	31	Tr	1	6	1
Potato chips, plain, salted, 8 oz.	1217	79	16	120	10
Potato salad, 1 cup	358	21	7	28	3
Potatoes, au gratin, 1 cup	323	19	12	28	4
Potatoes, baked, flesh, 1 potato	145	Tr	3	34	2
Potatoes, french fried, frozen, oven-heated, 10 strips	100	4	2	16	2
Pretzels, hard, salted, 10 twists	229	2	5	48	2

FOOD	CALORIES	FAT (g)	PROTEIN (g)	CARBS (g)	FIBER (g)
Prune juice, canned, 1 cup	182	Tr	2	45	3
Puddings, chocolate, ready-to-eat, 1 can (5 oz.)	197	6	4	33	1
Puddings, rice, ready-to-eat, 1 can (5 oz.)	231	11	3	31	Tr
Puddings, tapioca, ready-to-eat, 1 snack size (4 oz.)	134	4	2	22	Tr
Puddings, vanilla, ready-to-eat, 1 snack size (4 oz.)	146	4	3	25	0
Quinoa, cooked, 1 cup	636	10	22	117	10
Raisins, seedless, 1 oz. (60 raisins)	85	Tr	Tr	22	2
Raspberries, raw, 10 berries	10	Tr	Tr	2	1
Refried beans, canned, 1 cup	237	3	14	39	13
Rhubarb, raw, diced, 1 cup	26	Tr	1	6	2
Rib, eye, broiled, 3 oz.	174	8	25	0	0
Rib, prime, roasted, 3 oz.	361	31	18	0	0
Rice noodles, cooked, 1 cup	192	Tr	2	44	2
Rice, brown, long-grain, cooked, 1 cup	216	2	5	45	4
Rice, white, long-grain, cooked, 1 cup	205	Tr	4	45	1
Salad dressing, French, 1 tbsp	73	7	Tr	2	0
Salad dressing, Italian, 1 tbsp	43	4	Tr	2	0
Salad dressing, thousand island, 1 tbsp	59	6	Tr	2	Tr
Salad dressing, vinegar and oil, 1 tbsp	72	8	0	Tr	0
Salad, without dressing, ¾ cup	17	Tr	1	3	na
Salad, without dressing, with cheese and egg, 1 ½ cups	102	6	9	5	na
Salami, cooked, beef, 1 slice	67	6	3	Tr	0
Salmon, smoked (lox), 1 oz.	33	1	5	0	0
Salmon, sockeye, cooked, 3 oz.	184	9	23	0	0
Sardine, Atlantic, canned in oil, drained, 1 small	25	1	3	0	0
Sauce, barbecue, 8 fl. oz.	188	5	5	32	3
Sauce, cheese, ¼ cup	110	8	4	4	Tr
Sauce, pasta, spaghetti/marinara, 1 cup	143	5	4	21	4
Sauce, salsa, ½ cup	36	Tr	2	8	2
Sausage, Italian, pork, cooked, 1 link	268	21	17	1	0
Sausage, meatless, 1 link	64	5	5	2	1
Scallops, breaded/fried, 2 large	67	3	6	3	0
Semisweet chocolate chips, 1 cup (6 oz. package)	805	50	7	106	10

FOOD	CALORIES	FAT (g)	PROTEIN (g)	CARBS (g)	FIBER (g)
Sherbet, orange, ½ cup (4 fl. oz.)	107	1	1	22	2
Short loin, porterhouse steak, broiled, 3 oz.	280	22	19	0	0
Shrimp, 1 medium	6	Tr	1	Tr	0
Shrimp, breaded and fried, (6–8shrimp)	454	25	19	40	na
Skirt steak, broiled, 3 oz.	174	9	23	0	0
Snapper, cooked, 3 oz.	109	1	22	0	0
Soup, beef noodle, canned, 8 fl. oz.	83	3	5	9	1
Soup, black bean, canned, 1 cup	116	2	6	20	4
Soup, chicken noodle, canned, 8 fl. oz.	75	2	4	9	1
Soup, chicken vegetable, chunky, 8 fl. oz.	166	5	12	19	na
Soup, chicken with rice, canned, 8 fl. oz.	60	2	4	7	1
Soup, clam chowder, New England, canned, 1cup	164	7	9	17	1
Soup, cream of mushroom, canned, 8 fl. oz.	203	14	6	15	Tr
Soup, minestrone, canned, 8 fl. oz.	82	3	4	11	1
Soup, split pea with ham, chunky, 1 cup	185	4	11	27	4
Soup, tomato, canned, 8 fl. oz.	85	2	2	17	Tr
Soup, vegetable beef, canned, 8 fl. oz.	78	2	6	10	Tr
Soy milk, fluid, 1 cup	120	5	9	11	3
Spaghetti, cooked, 1 cup	197	1	7	40	2
Squash, winter, butternut, baked, cubes, 1 cup	82	Tr	2	22	na
Strawberries, whole, 1 cup	46	Tr	Tr	11	Tr
Sugar cookie	66	3	1	8	Tr
Sunflower seed kernels, dried, without hulls, 1 cup	821	71	33	27	15
Sweet potato, baked in skin, 1 medium	103	Tr	2	24	4
Sweet rolls, cinnamon, with raisins	223	10	4	31	1
Syrups, chocolate, fudge, 2 tbsp	133	3	2	24	1
Syrups, pancake, 1 tbsp	47	0	0	12	Tr
Taco salad, 1 ½ cups	279	15	13	24	na
Taco, 1 small	369	21	21	27	na
Tangerines, raw, 1 medium	37	Tr	1	9	2
Tea, brewed, 8 fl. oz.	2	0	0	1	0
Tempeh, 1 cup	320	18	31	16	na
Tenderloin, broiled, 3 oz.	247	17	21	0	0

FOOD	CALORIES	FAT (g)	PROTEIN (g)	CARBS (g)	FIBER (g)
Tofu, firm, prepared, ¼ block	62	4	7	2	Tr
Tomato juice, canned, with salt added, 1 cup	41	Tr	2	10	1
Tomato paste, canned, 1 cup	215	1	11	50	12
Tomato sauce, with vegetables, canned, 1 cup	103	2	2	22	4
Tomatoes, raw, 1 cup, chopped	32	Tr	2	7	2
Tomatoes, stewed, 1 cup	66	Tr	2	16	3
Tomatoes, sun-dried, packed in oil, drained, 1 cup	234	15	6	26	6
Tonic water, 12 fl. oz.	124	0	0	32	na
Tortilla chips, plain, 1 oz.	142	7	2	18	2
Trout, rainbow, wild, cooked, 3 oz.	128	5	19	0	0
Tuna, fresh, bluefin, cooked, 3 oz.	156	5	25	0	0
Tuna, light, canned in water, drained, 1 can	191	1	42	0	0
Tuna, white, canned in water, drained, 1 can	220	5	41	0	0
Turkey, breast, meat and skin, roasted, ½ breast	1633	64	248	0	0
Turkey, ground, cooked, 1 patty (4oz. raw)	193	11	22	0	0
Turkey, leg, meat and skin, roasted, 1 leg	1136	54	152	0	0
Veal, boneless breast, braised, 3 oz.	226	14	23	0	0
Veal, ground, broiled, 3 oz.	146	6	21	0	0
Vegetable juice cocktail, 1 cup	46	Tr	2	11	2
Vegetables, mixed, frozen, boiled, ½ cup	59	Tr	3	12	4
Waffle, plain, frozen	98	3	2	15	1
Walnuts, English, 7 nuts	183	18	4	4	2
Waterchestnuts, raw, sliced, ½ cup	60	Tr	1	15	2
Watermelon, raw, 1/16 of melon	86	Tr	2	22	1
Whipped cream, 1 tbsp	8	1	Tr	Tr	0
White Cake	264	9	4	42	1
Wild rice, cooked, 1 cup	166	1	7	35	3
Yogurt, fruit, low-fat, 8 fl. oz.	243	3	10	46	0
Yogurt, plain, nonfat, 8 fl. oz.	137	Tr	14	19	0
Yogurt, vanilla, low-fat, 8 fl. oz.	208	3	12	34	0

FOOD	CALORIES	FAT (g)	PROTEIN (g)	CARBS (g)	FIBER (g)

WEIGHT CHART

Chart your weight as you use this journal.

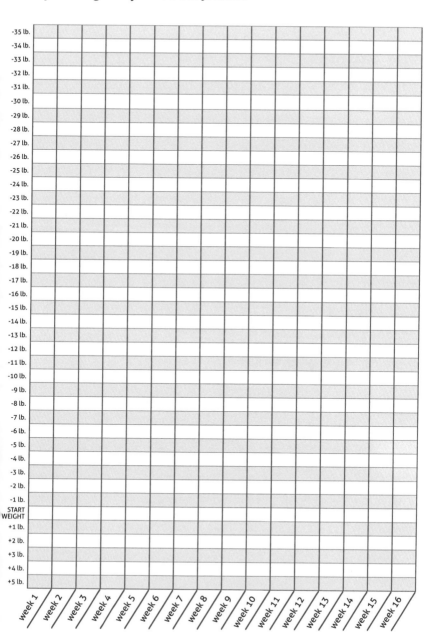

IN CLOSING

With this diet and fitness journal complete, please record any closing thoughts you may have.

Would you like to continue your weight loss journey?

_____

_____

_____

_____

_____

_____

_____

_____

Have you achieved your goals?

_____

_____

_____

_____

_____

_____

_____

_____

What have you learned from this process?

_____

_____

_____

_____

_____

_____

_____

_____

_____

_____

_____

_____

_____

_____

_____

_____

_____

_____

NOTES